How Well Do You Know Your Medications?

Prescription Drug Overdose Signs and Symptoms

Written by
Meridith Berk

Overdose:
Signs and Symptoms of Overdose for Top
Prescription Drugs

An **overdose** is when you take more than the normal or recommended amount of something, usually a drug. An overdose may result in serious, harmful symptoms or death. If the overdose happens by mistake, it is called an accidental overdose. When it is taken by the person intentionally it is called a suicide attempt or if successful, a suicide. Both of these occur far more frequently than you would think.

With the number and variety of drugs being prescribed these days it becomes extremely important to be aware not only of the side effects these medications can cause but the symptoms of overdose as well. Certain substances including the full spectrum of psychiatric drugs can be especially risky because the individual who is taking them may be unaware of the changes that are occurring in their physical state, personality and behavior. This is when it is most important for those around the patient to be fully aware of the side effects and overdose symptoms of those drugs so they can be aware if these start happening to a friend or loved-one. This knowledge and awareness can save lives.

The symptoms of overdose can sometimes be similar to the side effects listed for that particular drug. With any medication it is important to always err on the side of safety and caution. If you suspect problems from any drug even if no mention has been made of that reaction here or in any presentation of side effects, warnings or overdose symptoms call local emergency services at 911 and poison control. Don't take any chances. If you think you are having any other kind of adverse reaction to any drug or combination of drugs you're taking, call emergency medical services at 911.

This booklet only includes the overdose symptoms. All drugs also have side effects and other warnings. Some of these side effects are life threatening and the warnings vital so it is also important before taking a medication or allowing someone in your care to take one that you fully educate yourself on the side effects and warnings connected with a prescription drug.

Side Effect and Warnings for Pharmaceutical Drugs are available from MedlinePlus, a service of the National Library of Medicine and the National Institutes of Health.

http://www.nlm.nih.gov/medlineplus/druginformation.html

https://www.nlm.nih.gov/medlineplus/druginfo/drug_Aa.html

The number for the U.S. National Poison Hotline is 1-800-222-1222

In this booklet I'll be detailing the published commonly reported overdose symptoms for most of the best selling and most prescribed pharmaceutical drugs. Oddly enough the FDA MedlinePlus web site does not always list all the overdose symptoms that may be connected with a specific drug. Therefore I have gone to several sources to compile the most complete and accurate list of these symptoms that I can. (Sources are listed at the end of this publication).

Currently there are over 4,400 different prescription drugs available on the U.S. market. Not all of them can be found in these pages. Some of the drugs are not likely to be the cause of overdose, others are only available under strict control (such as those used in chemotherapy) and still others have come onto the market since the writing of this book.

If a medication you are taking is not included in here, information can be found by calling poison control or (if not an emergency) checking the three websites listed in bold at the very end of the book.

Brand name drugs will be listed first in alphabetical order. After the brand name drugs I've included a separate section where the drugs will be listed alphabetically by their generic or chemical name. In a few circumstances I have listed the generic name in both places to aid in finding the overdose information quickly

If you experience any of the following symptoms of drug overdose, call emergency services at 911 right away. If you think you may have taken too much of any drug or taken it with another drug or with alcohol which could be causing any negative effects call Emergency Services at 911 right away. You may experience overdose symptoms not included here.

If you become aware of a friend or loved one who is taking prescription medication experiencing or manifesting any of these symptoms call 911 immediately.

If possible, have the following information to hand:

Patient's age, weight and condition

Name of the medication (the ingredients and strengths, if known)

Time it was taken

Amount taken

If the medicine was prescribed for the patient
Any other medications, alcohol or other drugs the person has ingested

If you suspect you may have overdosed on any drug it is best to check with poison control right away, even if you do not have any symptoms. The people there have the experience and education to tell you what to do and if you need to contact emergency services at 911. The National Poison Control Center (1-800-222-1222) can be called from anywhere in the United States. This national hotline number will let you talk to experts in poisoning. You can call and ask questions at any time. It does not have to be an emergency.

Patient Rights and Informed Consent

Before I get into listing prescription medications with their overdose signs and symptoms, I'd like to add a note about Patient's Rights, Patient's Fredoms, and Informed Consent.

Patient's Rights, Patient's Freedoms and a Patient's Right to Informed Consent were all developed to protect the right of a patient within the healthcare environment. All three of these are written out here. However, the most important and the one that is legally binding is Informed Consent.

What is the Patient's Bill of Rights?

Here you will find a summary of the Consumer Bill of Rights and Responsibilities that was adopted by the US Advisory Commission on Consumer Protection and Quality in the Health Care Industry in 1998. It is also known as the Patient's Bill of Rights.

The Patient's Bill of Rights was created to try to reach 3 major goals:

1. To help patients feel more confident in the US health care system; the Bill ofRights:

• Assures that the health care system is fair and it works to meet patients' needs

• Gives patients a way to address any problems they may have

• Encourages patients to take an active role in staying or getting healthy

2. To stress the importance of a strong relationship between patients and their health care providers

3. To stress the key role patients play in staying healthy by laying out rights and responsibilities for all patients and health care providers

This Bill of Rights also applies to the insurance plans offered to federal employees. Many other health insurance plans and facilities have also adopted these values. Even Medicare and Medicaid stand by many of them.

The 8 key areas of the Patient's Bill of Rights

Information for patients

You have the right to accurate and easily-understood information about your health plan, health care professionals, and health care facilities. If you speak another language, have a physical or mental disability, or just don't understand something, help should be given so you can make informed health care decisions.

Choice of providers and plans

You have the right to choose health care providers who can give you high-quality health care when you need it.

Access to emergency services

If you have severe pain, an injury, or sudden illness that makes you believe that your health is in danger, you have the right to be screened and stabilized using emergency services. You should be able to use these services whenever and wherever you need them, without needing to wait for authorization and without any financial penalty.

Taking part in treatment decisions

You have the right to know your treatment options and take part in decisions about your care. Parents, guardians, family members, or others that you choose can speak for you if you cannot make your own decisions.

Respect and non-discrimination

You have a right to considerate, respectful care from your doctors, health plan representatives, and other health care providers that does not discriminate against you.

Confidentiality (privacy) of health information

You have the right to talk privately with health care providers and to have your health care information protected. You also have the right to read and copy your own medical records. You have the right to ask that your doctor change your record if it is not correct, relevant, or complete.

Complaints and appeals

You have the right to a fair, fast, and objective review of any complaint you have against your health plan, doctors, hospitals or other health care personnel. This includes complaints about waiting times, operating hours, the actions of health care personnel, and the adequacy of health care facilities.

Consumer responsibilities

In a health care system that protects consumer or patients' rights, patients should expect to take on some responsibilities to get well and/or stay well (for instance, exercising and not using tobacco). Patients are expected to do things like treat health care workers and other patients with respect, try to pay their medical bills, and follow the rules and benefits of their health plan coverage. Having patients involved in their care increases the chance of the best possible outcomes and helps support a high quality, cost-conscious health care system.

Patients Freedoms

The Association of American Physicians and
Surgeons adopted a list of patient freedoms in 1990, which
was modified and adopted as a 'patients' bill of rights' in
1995:

All patients should be guaranteed the following freedoms:

To seek consultation with the physician(s) of their choice;

To contract with their physician(s) on mutually agreeable
terms;

To be treated confidentially, with access to their records
limited to those involved in their care or designated by the
patient;

To use their own resources to purchase the care of their
choice;

To refuse medical treatment even if it is recommended by
their physician(s);

To be informed about their medical condition, the risks and
benefits of treatment and appropriate alternatives;

To refuse third-party interference in their medical care, and
to be confident that their actions in seeking or declining
medical care will not result in third-party-imposed
penalties for patients or physicians;

To receive full disclosure of their insurance plan in plain
language

A Patient's Right to Informed Consent

Too many patients get handed a prescription by their doctor without first being given enough information to decide for themselves whether they should take it. You may not know this, but your doctor has a legal as well as ethical obligation to explain to you your diagnosis as well as the benefits and potential risks associated with any medication he or she is prescribing.

In the current healthcare landscape, practitioners are under significant financial pressure to keep the time they spend with patients at a minimum. In the United States, the average doctor's appointment lasts less than 15 minutes. In the United Kingdom appointments are even shorter. This is barely enough time to find out what is bothering the person and do a minimal physical examination.

This limited time, however, is no excuse for dashing off a prescription without meeting the Informed Consent requirement.

We as patients, need to assume responsibility for our care by demanding our right to Informed Consent. If this means the appointment runs over its allotted time, so be it. Maybe the healthcare system will need to change to better allow for a real doctor-patient relationship and the true caring that implies.

What's Informed Consent?

The actual laws vary from state to state, but the bottom line is that a physician practicing in the United States must explain a diagnosis, as well as alternatives and potential risks of treatment to the patient or become potentially liable for negligence or even battery, depending on the circumstances. (Similar laws are in place in many other countries as well including Canada, Great Britain and Australia.)

Informed Consent regulations demand the information passed on to the patient be given in a way they understand. Naturally, this means the healthcare provider or a translator must communicate in a language the patient understands. That's obvious. But, how about relaying the data in terms understandable to those of us who don't have a medical degree? Too much information about potential risks can be hidden in incomprehensible (to the patient) medical terminology.

Here are the rules for Informed Consent:

The physician (not a delegated representative) should disclose and discuss:

The diagnosis, if known

The nature and purpose of a proposed treatment or procedure

The risks and benefits of proposed treatment or procedures Alternatives (regardless of costs or extent covered by insurance)

The risks and benefits of alternatives

The risks and benefits of not receiving treatments or undergoing procedures

The most important goal of informed consent is for the patient to have the opportunity to be an informed participant in his or her own care.

The informed consent process is an opportunity for patient and physician to work together in a cooperative effort to get the best care for *you*, the patient.

Resources:

Patient's Bill of Rights

Patient's Freedoms

Legal Dictionary

Prescription Medications and their Overdose Signs And Symptoms

First list is alphabetical by brand name. Second section is alphabetical by generic name.

Symptoms and signs of overdose may include but are not limited to...

Alphabetical by Brand Name

Abilify (aripiprazole)

Aggression
Agitation
Changes in heartbeat
Confusion
Coma
Difficulty breathing
Drowsiness
Fainting
Feeling light-headed
High blood pressure
Irregular heart rhythm
Lethargy (sleepy, drowsy, out of sorts, sluggish, apathetic –
it can also mean a state of unconsciousness resembling a
deep sleep)
Loss of consciousness
Low Blood Potassium (your doctor can test for this)
Movements you cannot control
Nausea
Pneumonia
Seizures
Shakiness
Slowed Heart Rate
Unusual mental changes
Vomiting
Weakness
Widened Pupils (the black circles in the middle of the eyes)

Actos (pioglitazone)

Since there have been very few reported cases of people
who have overdosed on Actos, the full effects of an Actos
overdose are not known. But any medication taking in
excess can cause serious problems. If you suspect you have
taken too much Actos do not wait for symptoms but call
poison control and 911 right away.

Adderall / Adderall XR
(dextroamphetamine and amphetamine salts)

An overdose of Adderall can be fatal. If you think you or
someone you know may have overdosed get help
immediately even if you are unaware of any symptoms.

Aggressiveness / Aggressive behavior
Behavior Changes
Blurred vision
Coma
Confusion
Convulsions
Dark red or cola-colored urine
Dehydration
Delusions
Depression
Diarrhea
Dizziness
Fainting
Fast heartbeats
Feeling light-headed
Feelings of panic
Fever or flu symptoms

Hallucinations (seeing things and hearing voices that do not exist)
Heart attack
Increased blood pressure
Lower abdominal pain
Muscle weakness
Muscle Twitches
Nausea
Numbness
Numbing of fingertips
Panic
Personality changes
Rapid breathing
Restlessness
Seizures (convulsions)
Stomach pain
Stroke
Sweating
Swelling of hands, feet or ankles
Tiredness
Tremor
Trouble concentrating
Uncontrollable shaking of a part of the body
Uneven or irregular heartbeats
Unexplained muscle pain or tenderness
Upset stomach
Vomiting
Weakness

Chronic abuse can manifest itself as psychosis

Advair Diskus (fluticasone and salmeterol)

Blurred vision
Chest pain
Difficulty falling or staying asleep
Dizziness
Dry mouth
Excessive tiredness
Fainting
Fast, pounding or irregular heartbeat
Headaches
Lack of energy
Muscle cramps or weakness
Nausea
Nervousness
Seizures
Shaking of a part of your body that you cannot control

Alprazolam (alprazolam)

Appearance of being drunk
Coma
Confusion
Coordination problems
Death
Difficulty breathing
Difficulty walking and talking
Dizziness
Drowsiness
Fainting
Feeling light-headed
Loss of balance or coordination
Muscle weakness
Problems with coordination
Sleepiness

Slow heartbeat
Slow reflexes

An overdose of alprazolam can be fatal. If you think you or someone you know may have overdosed get help immediately even if you are unaware of any symptoms.

Ambien / Ambien CR (zolpidem)
Coma
Confusion
Drowsiness
Fainting
Lightheadedness
Shallow breathing
Sleepiness
Slowed breathing
Slowed heartbeat

If you become aware of a friend or loved one who is taking prescription medication experiencing or manifesting any of these symptoms call 911 immediately. An overdose of Ambien can be fatal when it is taken together with other medications that can cause drowsiness.

Amoxil (amoxicillin)

Agitation
Behavior changes
Coma
Confusion
Loss of feeling in fingers or toes
Pain in fingers or toes
Pain or twitching
Seizure (black out or convulsions)

Severe skin rash
Urination changes (urinating less than you usually do)

Seek emergency medical attention right away if you think
you have overdosed on this medicine.

Anafranil (clomipramine)

Agitation
Blue discoloration of the skin
Blue lips or fingernails
Blurred vision
Cardiac arrest (heart attack)
Coma
Confusion
Congestive heart failure
Convulsions
Death
Drowsiness
Fainting
Fast or uneven heartbeat
Fever
Hallucinations
Kidney failure
Light-headedness
Loss of coordination
Low blood pressure (hypotension)
Muscle stiffness
Rapid heart rate (tachycardia)
Restlessness
Seizures
Shortness of breath
Slowed breathing
Stiff muscles
Severe Sweating

Swelling
Unusual body movements
Urination changes (urinating less or more than usual)
Vomiting
Widened pupils (the pupil is the dark circle in the center of the eye)

An overdose of Anafranil (clomipramine) can be fatal. If you think you or someone you know may have overdosed get help immediately even if you are unaware of any symptoms.

Aricept (donepezil)

Blurred vision
Collapse
Convulsions
Difficulty breathing
Dizziness (prolonged or severe)
Drooling
Extreme muscle weakness
Fainting
Feeling light-headed
Low blood pressure
Muscle weakness
Nausea
Salivation
Seizures
Severe nausea
Shallow breathing
Slow breathing
Slow heartbeat
Sweating
Vomiting
Watering mouth

Overdose with Aricept can be life threatening. If you suspect you have taken more than the prescribed amount of this medication call Emergency Services at 911.

Tenormin (atenolol)

Blurred vision
Breathing problems (slow or shallow breathing)
Chest pain
Confusion
Congestive heart failure (a life-threatening condition where the heart can no longer pump enough blood to the rest of the body)
Difficulty breathing
Dizziness
Fainting
Headache
Hunger (sudden hunger)
Lack of energy
Low blood sugar
Low blood pressure
Numbness or tingling of the mouth
Pale color
Pounding in chest
Rapid heartbeat
Seizures
Severe dizziness
Severe weakness
Slow heartbeat
Sluggishness
Sweating
Tiredness (excessive)
Very slow heartbeat (unusually slow heartbeat)
Weakness
Wheezing

Ativan (lorazepam)

Appearance of being drunk
Breathing difficulty
Coma
Confusion
Difficulty talking
Drowsiness
Extreme drowsiness
Fainting
Hypnotic state
Low blood pressure
Mental confusion
Muscle weakness
Reduced muscle tone
Shallow breathing
Sleepiness
Slow heart beat
Stupor
Tiredness
Unsteady walk
Weakness

Avandia (rosaglitizone)

Coma
Confusion
Convulsions
Dizziness
Drowsiness
Fainting
Hunger
Irritability
Low blood surag
Rapid Heartbeat (tachycardia)

Seizure
Sweating
Tremors
Weakness

Avastin (bevacizumab injection)

Severe headache

Avodart (dutasteride)

An overdose of Avodart is not expected to produce life-threatening symptoms.

Boniva (ibandronate)

Convulsions
Diarrhea
Heartburn
Indigestion
Irritability
Muscle cramps
Nausea
Numbness
Seizure
Stomach pain
Tight muscles in your face
Tingling
Ulcers
Unusual thoughts or behavior

BuSpar (buspirone)

Blurred vision
Dizziness
Drowsiness
Nausea
Stomach pain
Unusually small pupils
Upset stomach
Very deep sleep
Vomiting

Caduet (atorvastatin and amlodipine)

Dizziness
Fainting
Feeling light-headed
Rapid heartbeat
Redness
Severe warmth
Tingly feeling
Tingly under your skin

Carbatrol (carbamazepine)

Abnormal movements
Blurred vision
Difficulty urinating (urinating less or not at all)
Dizziness
Drowsiness
Fainting
Fast heartbeat

Feeling light-headed
Irregular or slowed breathing
Muscle twitching
Nausea
Rapid or pounding heartbeat
Restlessness
Shaking of a part of your body that you cannot control
Shallow breathing
Seizures
Slurred speech
Staggering walk
Tremors
Unconsciousness
Unsteadiness
Vomiting

Catapres (clonidine)

Anxiety
Blurred vision
Buzzing in your ears
Chest pain
Cold feeling
Cold, pale skin
Coma
Confusion
Decreased reflexes
Difficulty breathing
Drowsiness
Fainting
Feeling light-headed
High blood pressure
High blood pressure followed by low blood pressure
Irritability
Low blood pressure

Low body temperature
Seizures
Severe headache
Shallow or slow breathing
Shivering
Shortness of breath
Slow heart rate
Slurred speech
Smaller pupils - also called Pinpoint pupils (black circles in the middle of your eyes)
Tiredness
Weakness

Celexa (citlopram)

Amnesia (memory loss)
Blue skin
Coma
Confusion
Death
Dizziness
Drowsiness
Memory loss
Muscle pain
Nausea
Rapid breathing
Rapid, irregular or pounding heartbeat
Seizures
Sweating
Tremor (Shakiness)
Trouble breathing
Uncontrollable shaking of a part of the body
Vomiting

Chantix (varenicline)

Very little information is available about overdose symptoms related to Chantix, probably because it is relatively new on the market. Since it is reasonable to expect that some overdose symptoms could be related to the usual side effects connected to this drug I will list the side effects here.

Agitation
Appetite changes (increased or decreased appetite)
Bad taste in mouth
Behavior changes
Blistering of any kind of skin rash (Report to doctor immediately – no matter how mild)
Constipation
Depression
Difficulty breathing
Drowsiness
Fever
Gas
Headache
Heartburn
Hives
Hostility
Increased appetite
Indigestion
Mood changes
Nausea
Rash
Red skin
Skin rash
Sore throat
Stomach pain
Swelling of your face, lips, tongue or throat

Thoughts of suicide
Thoughts of hurting yourself
Tired feeling
Trouble falling asleep
Trouble staying asleep
Unpleasant taste in your mouth
Unusual dream or nightmares
Weakness
Vomiting

This is not a complete list of side effects, others may occur.

Cialis (tadalafil)

Chest Pain
Erection that lasts longer than 4 hours
Fainting
Feeling light-headed
Flushing
Headache
Heartburn
Indigestion
Irregular heartbeat
Nausea
Pain in the back
Pain in the muscles or any limb
Stuffy or runny nose

Clozaril (clozapine)

If overdose is suspected if even the symptoms are not on this list get to an emergency room immediately.

Change in heartbeat
Coma
Delerium
Difficult or slow breathing
Dizziness
Drowsines
Excessive salivation
Fainting
Fast or irregular heartbeat
Loss of consciousness
Seizures
Slow breathing
Severe or persistent dizziness
Severe or persistent drowsiness

Concerta (methylphenidate)

Aggressiveness
Agitation
Blurred vision
Confusion
Dry mouth and nose
Fainting
Fast breathing
Fast heartbeat
Fast, pounding or irregular heartbeat
Fever
Flushing
Hallucinations (seeing or hearing things that are not really there)

Headache
Hyperactivity (trouble sitting still)
Inappropriate happiness
Large pupils
Loss of consciousness
Muscle pains
Muscle twitches
Seizures (convulsions)
Shakiness
Sweating
Tremors
Uncontrollable shaking of a body part
Widening of pupils (the black circles in the middle of your eyes)
Vomiting

Crestor (rosuvastatin)

No specific information is available regarding overdose symptoms connected with taking Crestor. As with any other medication if you suspect you have taken an overdose of Crestor seek medical attention immediately.

Cymbalta (duloxetine)

Agitation
Coma
Confusion
Diarrhea
Dizziness
Drowsiness
Fainting
Fast heartbeat

Fever
Hallucinating (seeing things or hearing voices that do not exist)
Hypertension abnormally high blood pressure)
Hypotension (abnormally low blood pressure)
Light-headedness
Loss of coordination
Nausea
Seizures
Somnolence
Unresponsiveness
Vomiting

Depakene (valproic acid)

Coma
Confusion
Death
Decreased breathing
Deep Sleep
Drowsiness
Faint or no heartbeat
Heart block (a problem with the electrical system of the heart)
Irregular heartbeat
Loss of consciousness
Seizures
Shallow breathing
Sleepiness
Stopped breathing
Unconsciousness
Weak pulse

Depakote (valproic acid)

Coma
Confusion
Death
Decreased breathing
Deep Sleep
Drowsiness
Faint or no heartbeat
Heart block (a problem with the electrical system of the heart)
Irregular heartbeat
Loss of consciousness
Seizures
Shallow breathing
Sleepiness
Stopped breathing
Unconsciousness
Weak pulse

Desyrel (trazodone)

Breathing problems (breathing that slows or stops)
Changes in heartbeat
Death
Difficulty breathing
Drowsiness
Fast or pounding heartbeat
Irregular heart rhythm
Nausea
Priapism (a painful erection of the penis that does not go away)
Seizures
Vomiting

An overdose of trazodone can be fatal when it is taken with alcohol, barbiturates such as phenobarbital, or sedatives such as diazepam (Valium).

Dexedrine (dextroamphetamine)

Abdominal cramps
Aggressive behavior
Blurred Vision
Coma
Confusion
Convulsions
Depression
Diarrhea
Dizziness
Fainting
Fast breathing
Fatigue
Feeling light-headed
Fever
Flu symptoms
Hallucinations (seeing things or hearing voices that do not exist)
Heart rhythm abnormalities
Hyperactivity
Increased reflexes
Irregular heartbeat
Muscle pain
Muscle twitches
Muscle weakness or aching
Nausea
Panic
Rapid breathing
Restlessness
Seizures

Stomach cramps
Tiredness
Tremor
Uncontrollable shaking of a part of your body
Uneven heartbeats
Upset stomach
Urine changes (dark red or cola colored urine)
Vomiting
Weakness

An overdose of dextroamphetamine can be fatal.

Effexor / Effexor XR (venlafaxine)

Blurred vision
Burning of hands and feet
Cold spells
Coma
Convulsions
Death
Decreased blood pressure
Dizziness
Drowsiness
Excessive tiredness (somnolence)
Hot spells
Increased heart rate
Increased size of pupil (black center of the eye)
Irregular heartbeats
Liver damage
Muscle Pain
Nausea
Numbness
Numbness of hands and feet
Seizures
Sleepiness

Slowed heart rate
Spinning sensation (vertigo)
Tingling of hands and feet
Unconsciousness
Vomiting

Elavil (amitriptyline)

Agitation
Blurred vision
Changes in heart rhythm
Cold body temperature
Coma
Confusion
Convulsions
Drowsiness
Fainting
Feeling cold
Feeling hot
Feeling light-headed
Fever
Hallucinating (seeing things or hearing voices that do not exist)
Hypotension (very low blood pressure)
Irregular heartbeats
Muscle stiffness
Problems concentrating
Restlessness
Rigid muscles
Seizures
Sleepiness
Sweating
Uneven heartbeats
Vomiting

An overdose of Elavil can be fatal.

Enbrel (etanercept injection)

No harmful effects due to large doses of etanercept (Enbrel) have been reported. However if you suspect you have been given too much of this drug notify your doctor right away.

Epogen (epoetin alfa injection)

Blood clot in hemodialysis port (Hemodialysis is the removal of toxins or waste from the kidneys. Medically, a port is a small device used to put something into the body placed below the skin or in a vein)

Blue-grey color or darkening around mouth or nails
Chest pain (squeezing pressure or tightness)
Cough that won't go away
Coughing up blood
Discomfort or pain in the arms, shoulder, neck, jaw and back
Dizziness
Excessive sweating
Extreme tiredness
Extreme weakness
Fainting or loss of consciousness
Fullness in your upper stomach
Fast or irregular heartbeat
Headache (sudden and severe)
Increased blood pressure
Itching (especially after bathing)
Leg pain, tenderness, redness, warmth and / or swelling
Light-headedness

Loss of balance or coordination
Redness of the face
Seizure
Shortness of breath
Sudden confusion
Sudden trouble seeing in one or both eyes
Sudden trouble speaking or understanding speech
Sudden weakness or numbness of an arm or a leg
(especially on one side of the body)
Sudden weakness or numbness of the face (especially one side)
Swelling of hands, feet, or ankles
Trouble walking (sudden)
Vision problems

Eskalith (lithium carbonate)

Blurred vision
Confusion
Convulsions
Diarrhea
Drowsiness
Increased thirst
Increased urine output
Loss of appetite
Loss of coordination
Low blood pressure
Muscle twitching
Muscle weakness
Nausea
Rash
Ringing in your ears
Seizures
Sluggishness
Tremor

Vomiting

Evista (raloxifene)

Coordination problems
Diarrhea
Dizziness
Flushing
Leg cramps
Loss of coordination
Rash
Shakiness
Tremor
Vomiting

Flomax (tamsulosin)

Blurred vision
Cold and clammy skin
Coma
Dizziness
Extreme dizziness
Fainting
Headache
Light-headedness
Loss of consciousness
Upset stomach
Weak, fast pulse
Weakness

Furosemide (furosemide)

Confusion
Dizziness
Fainting
Fatigue
Feeling light-headed
Irregular pulse
Loss of appetite
Muscle cramps
Nausea
Ringing in your ears
Vomiting
Weakness

Geodon (ziprasidone)

Anxiety
Dizziness
Drowsiness
Fainting
Fast or pounding heartbeat
Feeling light-headed
Fever
High blood pressure (hypertension)
Increased heart rate
Irregular heart rhythms
Muscle spasms
Problems with speech
Restless muscle movements in your eyes
Restless muscle movements in your tongue jaw or neck
Shakiness
Slurred speech
Sudden movements that you cannot control
Sweating

Twitching
Uncontrollable movements of the arms, hands or tongue
Uncontrollable shaking of a part of the body
Unusual body movements

Glocophage (metformin)

An overdose of metformin (Glucophage) can be life-threatening. If you suspect an overdose has occurred get emergency help immediately.

An overdose of metformin may cause a life-threatening condition called lactic acidosis. Get emergency medical help if you have any of these symptoms of lactic acidosis: weakness, increasing sleepiness, slow heart rate, cold feeling, muscle pain, shortness of breath, stomach pain, feeling light-headed, and fainting.

Other overdose signs and symptoms include:

Abnormally fast or slow heartbeat
Blurry vision
Cold sweats
Coma
Confusion
Convulsions
Death
Decreased appetite
Deep, rapid breathing
Difficulty speaking
Discomfort
Dizziness
Drowsiness
Extreme tiredness

Fainting
Feeling cold
Flushing of the skin
Headache
Hunger
Irritability
Light-headedness
Loss of consciousness
Loss of coordination
Muscle pain
Nausea
Shakiness
Shortness of breath
Seizures
Stomach pain
Sweating
Tremors
Vomiting
Weakness

Haldol (haloperidol)

An overdose of haloperidol can be fatal.

Arrhythmia (an irregular heart rhythm)
Coma
Difficulty breathing
Drowsiness
Extreme drowsiness
Feeling like you might pass out
Loss of consciousness
Low blood pressure (hypotension)
Muscle weakness
Rigid muscles
Shakiness

Sleepiness
Slowed breathing
Stiff or weak muscles
Tremors
Uncontrolled muscle movements in your eyes
Uncontrolled muscle movements in your tongue, jaw or neck
Unusual, slowed or uncontrollable movements of any part of the body

Hydrochlorothiazide

Back pain
Confusion
Decreased urine output
Dehydration
Diarrhea
Dizziness
Drowsiness
Dry mouth
Extremely low blood pressure
Fainting
Fatigue
Headache
Increased thirst
Increased urination
Kidney Failure
Lethargy
Lightheadedness
Loss of Consciousness
Muscle pain or cramps
Muscle weakness
Nausea
Restlessness
Seizures

Slow or irregular heartbeat
Tiredness
Thirst
Weakness
Unconsciousness
Vomiting

Intuniv (guanfacine)

Accidental **overdose** of **Guanfacine** is an increasing cause of poisoning in children 3 years of age and younger. (From Drugs.com)

Blurred vision
Difficult breathing
Dizziness
Drowsiness
Drowsiness leading to unresponsiveness or coma
Fainting
Feeling like you might pass out
Irritability
Lack of energy
Lightheadedness
Nausea
Seizures (possibly)
Slowed breathing
Slowed heart rate
Sluggish feeling
Smaller pupils (black circles in the middle of the eyes)
Vomiting
Weakness

Januvia (sitagliptin)

Agitation
Coma
Confusion
Convulsions
Dizziness
Drowsiness
Fainting
Fast heartbeat
Headache
Hunger (as a sign of low blood sugar)
Irritability
Seizures
Sweating
Tremors
Vision changes
Weakness
If you think you may have taken more than the prescribed amount of Januvia seek emergency medical attention right away.

Klonopin (clonazepam)

Alterations in mental status
Appearance of being drunk
Coma
Confusion
Difficulty breathing
Difficulty talking
Difficulty walking
Diminished reflexes
Dizziness
Drowsiness

Fainting
Muscle weakness
Slow heartbeat
Somnolence (a state of sleepiness, drowsiness)

If you suspect you suspect you have taken an overdose of
this medication seek emergency medical attention right
away. In some circumstances, especially when this drug is
mixed with alcohol or other sedating drugs, overdose can
lead to the person being unable to breathe and dying.

Klonopin can be habit-forming and can lose its
effectiveness as you build a tolerance to it. This can lead to
unintentional overdose.

Lamictal (lamatrigine)

Arrhythmia (irregular heartbeat)
Blurred vision
Coma
Coordination problems
Crossed eyes
Death
Fainting
Feeling light-headed
Headache
Increased seizures
Involuntary eye movements
Loss of balance or coordination
Loss of consciousness
Seizures
Unconsciousness

Lasix (furosemide)

Confusion
Dizziness
Drowsiness
Fainting
Fatigue
Feeling light-headed
Irregular pulse
Loss of appetite
Muscle cramps
Muscle pain
Nausea
Ringing in your ears
Vomiting
Weak or irregular heartbeat
Weakness

Lexapro (escitalopram)

Coma
Confusion
Convulsions
Dizziness
Drowsiness
Fast breathing
Fast pounding heartbeat
Forgetfulness
Increased heart rate (tachycardia)
Insomnia
Irregular heart rhythm (arrhythmia)
Low blood pressure (hypotension)
Nausea
Rapid heartbeat (tachycardia)

Seizures
Sweating
Tremor

Lipitor (atorvastatin)

The symptoms of Lipitor overdose are not known. If you suspect you have taken more Lipitor than prescribed call poison control or your doctor right away.

Lisinopril (Prinvil, Zestril)

Dizziness
Extreme dizziness
Fainting
Fatigue
Light-headedness
Weakness

Lithium (lithium carbonate)

Blurred vision
Confusion
Convulsions
Diarrhea
Drowsiness
Increased thirst
Increased urine output
Loss of appetite
Loss of coordination
Low blood pressure
Muscle twitching
Muscle weakness

Nausea
Rash
Ringing in your ears
Seizures
Sluggishness
Tremor
Vomiting

Lithobid (lithium carbonate)

Blurred vision
Confusion
Convulsions
Diarrhea
Drowsiness
Increased thirst
Increased urine output
Loss of appetite
Loss of coordination
Low blood pressure
Muscle twitching
Muscle weakness
Nausea
Rash
Ringing in your ears
Seizures
Sluggishness
Tremor
Vomiting

Ludiomil (maprotiline)

Agitation
Blue fingernails
Blue lips
Confusion
Convulsions
Dizziness
Drowsiness (extreme)
Extreme drowsiness
Fast heart rate
Fever
Irregular heartbeat
Large pupils
Muscle weakness
Muscle stiffness
Poor memory
Restlessness
Seizures
Trouble breathing
Vomiting

Lunesta (eszopiclone)

A Lunesta overdose can be fatal.

Exceeding the prescribed dosage of Lunesta increases the risk of experiencing abnormal thoughts and engaging in reckless behavior. Examples include aggressive behaviors, confusion, increase in outgoingness, and suicidal ideation. In severe cases, coma and death may result.

Aggressive behaviors
Coma
Confusion
Death
Drowsiness
Increase in outgoingness
Reckless behavior
Suicidal ideation (thoughts of killing yourself)

Luvox (fluvoxamine)

Agitation
Blurred vision
Breathing problems
Cardiac problems (heart problems)
Coma
Convulsions
Death
Diarrhea
Dizziness
Drowsiness
Enlarged pupils
Extreme drowsiness
Fainting
Fast hear rate
Hyperactivity
Irregular heart rhythms (arrhythmias)
Lack of coordination
Liver function problems
Low blood pressure (hypotension)
Low blood potassium levels (hypokalemia)
Nausea

Rapid heart rate (tachycardia)
Seizures
Shakiness
Slowed heart rate (bradycardia)
Somnolence (drowsiness, sleepiness)
Tremors
Trouble breathing
Vomiting

Lyrica (pregabalin)

It is unknown exactly what to expect from a **Lyrica overdose**, but patients who are suspected of **overdosing** should seek emergency medical attention or contact the local Poison Control Center by calling 1-800-222-1222 or call local emergency services at 911.

Mellaril (thioridazine)

An overdose of Mellaril (methylphenidate) can be fatal. If you suspect an overdose, seek medical help immediately.

Agitation
Blurred vision
Coma
Confusion
Constipation
Convulsions
Decreased urination
Difficulty breathing
Difficulty urinating
Difficulty walking
Drooling

Drowsiness
Dry mouth
Dry skin
Extreme dizziness
Fainting
Fast heartbeat
Feeling hot or feeling cold
Fever
High body temperature
Intestinal obstruction
Irregular heartbeat (arrhythmias)
Loss of appetite
Loss of coordination
Low blood pressure (hypotension)
Low body temperature
Menstrual changes
Muscle spasms
Muscle stiffness
Narrowed pupil (black circle in the middle of each eye)
Nasal congestion
Pounding heartbeat
Rapid heart rate (tachycardia)
Restlessness
Seizures
Shallow breathing
Skin discoloration (blue to purple)
Slowed breathing
Slow heartbeat (bradycardia)
Slowed or unusual movements
Stiff neck or face
Stomach bloating
Stomach cramps
Stuffed nose
Swallowing difficulties
Ulcers in mouth, tongue or throat
Uncontrollable muscle movements

Vision color changes (things getting a brown tinge)
Weak breathing
Widened pupils (black circle in the middle of each eye)
Yellow eyes

Metadate (methylphenidate)

Aggressiveness
Agitation
Blurred vision
Confusion
Dry mouth and nose
Fainting
Fast breathing
Fast heartbeat
Fast, pounding or irregular heartbeat
Fever
Flushing
Hallucinations (seeing or hearing things that are not really there)
Headache
Hyperactivity (trouble sitting still)
Inappropriate happiness
Large pupils
Loss of consciousness
Muscle pains
Muscle twitches
Seizures (convulsions)
Shakiness
Sweating
Tremors
Uncontrollable shaking of a body part
Widening of pupils (the black circles in the middle of your eyes)
Vomiting

Methelyn (methylphenidate)

Aggressiveness
Agitation
Blurred vision
Confusion
Dry mouth and nose
Fainting
Fast breathing
Fast heartbeat
Fast, pounding or irregular heartbeat
Fever
Flushing
Hallucinations (seeing or hearing things that are not really there)
Headache
Hyperactivity (trouble sitting still)
Inappropriate happiness
Large pupils
Loss of consciousness
Muscle pains
Muscle twitches
Seizures (convulsions)
Shakiness
Sweating
Tremors
Uncontrollable shaking of a body part
Widening of pupils (the black circles in the middle of your eyes)
Vomiting

Moban (molindone)

Seek emergency medical attention immediately if you think you have used too much of this drug.

Agitation
Coma
Convulsions
Death
Difficulty breathing
Dizziness
Drowziness
Fainting
Fever
Increased salivation
Irregular heart rhythm (arrhythmia)
Loss on consciousness
Low blood pressure (hypotension)
Muscle stiffness
Muscle twitching
Restlessness
Seizures
Slurred speech
Trouble swallowing
Unconsciousness
Unusual body or facial movements
Unusual, slowed or uncontrollable movements of any part of the body

Nasonex (mometasone nasal inhalation)

An overdose of this medication is not likely to occur. If you do suspect an overdose contact poison control.

Nasonex is a topical steroid and long-term use of high steroid doses can lead to symptoms such as thinning skin, easy bruising, changes in the shape or location of body fat (especially in your face, neck, back, and waist), increased acne or facial hair, menstrual problems, impotence, or loss of interest in sex.

Neulasta (pegfilgrastim)

Overdose symptoms for this drug are not known.

Nexium (esomeprazole)

Blurred vision
Confusion
Drowsiness
Dry mouth
Fast heartbeat
Flushing
Headache
Increased heart rate (tachycardia)
Loss of coordination
Nausea
Seizures
Shortness of breath
Sweating
Tremor

Norpramin (desipramine)

An overdose of desipramine (Norpramin) can be fatal.

Agitation
Blurred vision
Change in heart rhythm
Coma
Confusion
Convulsions
Death
Dilated (wide open) pupils (the dark circle in the middle of
each eye)
Disturbed concentration
Drowsiness
Extremely low blood pressure
Feeling cold
Feeling hot
Hallucinations (seeing or hearing things that do not exist)
High fever
Irregular heart rate
Low body temperature (hypothermia)
Muscle stiffness
Muscle tension
Overactive reflexes
Rigid muscles
Seizures
Stupor
Trouble concentrating
Uneven heartbeats
Very low blood pressure
Vomiting

Orap (pimozide)

Blank facial expression
Coma
Death
Difficulty breathing
Dizziness
Drowsiness
Fast heartbeat
Restlessness
Shuffling walk
Uncontrollable movements
Unusual, slowed or uncontrollable movement of any part of the body

An overdose of Orap (pimozide) can be fatal.

Oxycontin (oxycodone)

Blue color of skin, fingernals, lips, area around the mouth
Cardiac arrest (heart attack)
Cold, clammy skin
Coma
Confusion
Death
Difficulty breathing
Dizziness
Excessive sleepiness
Extreme drowsiness, leading to coma
Fainting
Increase in size (dilated) of pupils (the black circles in the middle of the eye)
Loss of consciousness
Low blood pressure (hypotension)

Seizures
Shallow breathing
Slow breathing
Slowed or stopped breathing
Slow heart rate (bradycardia)
Small pupils (the black circles in the middle of the eye)
Tiredness
Weak, limp muscles
Weakness

An overdose of Oxycontin (oxycodone) can be fatal.

Pamelor (nortriptyline)

Agitation
Blurred vision
Confusion
Coma
Convulsions
Dilated pupils (the pupils are the dark circles in the middle of the eyes)
Disturbed concentration
Dizziness
Drowsiness
Excessive reflexes
Extreme drowsiness
Extremely high fever
Fainting
Fatigue
Feeling hot
Feeling cold
Fever
Fluid in the lungs
Hallucinations (seeing or hearing things that do not exist)
Heart failure

Irregular heartbeat
Low blood pressure
Low body temperature
Restlessness
Rigid muscles
Seizures
Shock
Stiff muscles
Stupor
Vomiting
Widened pupils (the pupils are the dark circles in the
middle of the eyes)

An overdose of nortriptyline can be fatal.

Parnate (tranylcypromine)

Agitation
Anxiety
Anxiousness
Chest pain
Cold sweats
Coma
Confusion
Dizziness
Drowsiness
Excitement
Fainting
Fast or pounding heart beat
Fatigue
Feeling light-headed
Fever
Flushing
Hallucinations (seeing or hearing things that do not exist)
Headache

High blood pressure (hypertension)
High fever
Hyperactivity
Insomnia (difficulty falling or staying asleep)
Irritability
Muscle twitching
Neck pain or stiffness
Restlessness
Sweating
Steffness
Twitching
Unclear speech
Very low blood pressure (hypotension)
Weakness

Paxil (paroxetine)

Aggressive behavior
Agitation
Blurred vision
Coma
Confusion
Dark red or brown urine
Death
Decreased urination
Diarrhea
Difficulty urinating
Difficulty walking
Dizziness
Drowsiness
Enlarged pupils
Extreme tiredness
Fainting
Fast, pounding, irregular, or slow heartbeat
Fever

Flu-like symptoms
Frenzied, abnormally excited mood
High blood pressure (hypertension)
Hyperactivity
Irregular heart rhythm (arrhythmia)
Kidney failure
Lack of energy
Liver problems, including hepatitis
Loss of appetite
Low blood pressure (hypotension)
Muscle pain, stiffness, or weakness
Nausea
Pain in the upper right part of the stomach
Rapid heartbeat (tachycardia)
Seizures
Shakiness
Slow heart rate (bradycardia)
Sudden muscle twitching or jerking that you cannot control
Sweating
Tremor
Uncontrollable shaking of a part of the body
Unusual bruising or bleeding
Vomiting
Yellowing of the skin and eyes

An overdose of Paxil can be fatal.

Plavix (clopidogrel)

Blood in your stools
Blood in your vomit
Difficulty breathing
Exhaustion
Shortness of breath
Unusual bruising or bleeding
Vomiting

Pristiq (desvenlafaxine)

Abdominal pain
Agitation
Constipation
Diarrhea
Dizziness
Drowsiness
Dry Mouth
Fast heartbeat (tachycardia)
Headache
Nausea
Numbness
Pain, burning, numbness or tingling in any part of the body
Seizures
Slow heart rate
Tingly Feeling
Tremor
Unusual sensations, such as burning or tingling
Vomiting

Prozac (fluoxetine)

Agitation
Coma
Confusion
Death
Drowsiness
Enlarged pupils
Fainting
Fast heart rate (tachycardia)
Fever
Hallucinating (seeing things or hearing voices other people don't)
High blood pressure (hypertension)

Hyperactivity
Irregular heart rhythm (arrhythmia)
Low blood pressure (hypotension)
Nausea
Nervousness
Pounding heart beat
Seizures
Sleepiness
Tremor
Uncontrollable shaking of part of the body
Uneven heartbeat
Unresponsiveness
Unsteadiness
Vomiting

Note: Possible overdose symptoms of Prozac include death.

Reclast   (zoledronic acid)

Confusion
Depression
Difficulty breathing
Difficulty speaking
Difficulty walking
Dizziness
Double vision
Fast, pounding or irregular heartbeat
Fever
Muscle stiffness
Muscle weakness
Numbness, burning or tingling in fingers or toes
Seizures
Shortness of breath
Spasms in the muscles of your face or other areas
Sudden tightening of muscles

Trouble breathing
Uneven heartbeats
Weakness
Wheezing

Remeron (mirtazapine)

Confusion
Death
Disorientation
Drowsiness
Memory problems
Poor memory
Rapid heart rate (tachycardia)
Note: Possible overdose symptoms of Remeron include death.

Remicade (infliximab)

An overdose of Remicade is not expected to produce life-threatening symptoms.

Risperdal (risperidone)

Blurred vision
Death
Dizziness
Drowsiness
Fainting
Fast, pounding or irregular heartbeat
Feeling light-headed
Fever
Irregular heart rhythm
Muscle spasms

Restless muscle movements in your eyes, tongue, jaw or neck
Seizures
Shakiness
Sweating
Uncontrollable movements of the arms, hands eyes, tongue, jaw or neck
Uncontrollable muscle contractions or other unusual body movements
Upset stomach
Note: Possible overdose symptoms of Risperdal (Risperidone) include death.

Ritalin (methylphenidate)

Aggressiveness
Agitation
Blurred vision
Confusion
Dry mouth and nose
Fainting
Fast breathing
Fast heartbeat
Fast, pounding or irregular heartbeat
Fever
Flushing
Hallucinations (seeing or hearing things that others do not)
Headache
Hyperactivity (trouble sitting still)
Inappropriate happiness
Large pupils
Loss of consciousness
Muscle pains
Muscle twitches
Seizures (convulsions)

Shakiness
Sweating
Tremors
Uncontrollable shaking of a body part
Widening of pupils (the black circles in the middle of your eyes)
Vomiting

Sarafem (fluoxetine)

Agitation
Coma
Confusion
Death
Drowsiness
Enlarged pupils
Fainting
Fast heart rate (tachycardia)
Fever
Hallucinating (seeing things or hearing voices other people don't)
High blood pressure (hypertension)
Hyperactivity
Irregular heart rhythm (arrhythmia)
Low blood pressure (hypotension)
Nausea
Nervousness
Pounding heart beat
Seizures
Sleepiness
Tremor
Uncontrollable shaking of part of the body
Uneven heartbeat
Unresponsiveness
Unsteadiness

Vomiting
Note: Possible overdose symptoms of Sarafem include death.

Seroquel (quetiapine)

Coma
Death
Dizziness
Drowsiness
Extreme Drowsiness
Fainting
Fast heartbeat (tachycardia)
Feeling light-headed
Irregular heart rhythm (arrhythmia)
Low blood potassium (hypokalemia)
Low blood pressure (hypotension)

Note: Possible overdose symptoms of Seroquel include death.

Singulair (montelukast)

Agitation
Dizziness
Headache
restlessness
Sleepiness
Stomach pain
Thirst
Vomiting

Stelazine (trifluoperazine)

Agitation
Bloating (of stomach)
Changes in heart rate
Coma
Constipation
Convulsions
Dizziness
Drowsiness
Dry mouth
Extreme drowsiness
Fainting
Fever
High body temperature
Intestinal blockage
Irregular heartbeat (arrhythmia)
Loss of consciousness
Low blood pressure (hypotension)
Low body temperature
Restlessness
Seizures
Severe Dizziness
Sleepiness
Stomach cramps
Uncontrollable movements
Unusual body movements
Slowed or uncontrollable movements of any part of the body
Very deep sleep

Strattera (atomoxetine)

Abnormal behavior
Agitation
Blurred vision
Dilated (wide) pupils (the drak circles in the center of each
eye)
Drowsiness
Dry mouth
Fast heart rate
Hallucinations (seeing or hearing things others do not)
Hyperactivity
Increase in activity or talking
Irregular heart rhythms (arrhythmias)
Sleepiness
Stomach or intestinal problems
Unusual behavior

Surmontil (trimipramine)

Abnormal dilation of the pupil (dark circle in the center of
each eye)
Agitation
Blurred vision
Changes in heart rhythm (arrhythmia)
Coma
Confusion
Convulsions
Death
Difficulty talking or articulating words
Dizziness
Drowsiness
Excitement
Extreme drowsiness
Fainting

Fatigue
Feeling light-headed
Hallucinations (seeing or hearing things that so not exist)
High fever
Low blood pressure (hypotension)
Low body temperature (hypothermia)
Muscle spasms
Muscle stiffness or tension
Seizures
Trouble breathing
Trouble concentrating
Uneven heartbeats
Vomiting
Note: An overdose of Surmontil (trimipramine) can be fatal

Symbicort (budesonide and fomoterol)

Cardiac arrest (heart attack)
Chest pain
Convulsions
Death
Difficulty falling asleep or staying asleep
Dizziness
Dry mouth
Excessive tiredness
Fainting
Fast, pounding or irregular heartbeat
Fatigue
Headache
Heart palpitations (feeling of a rapidly or forcefully beating heart)
High blood pressure (hypertension)
High blood sugar (hyperglycemia)
Increased salivation
Low blood pressure (hypotension)

Low blood potassium (hypokalemia)
Muscle cramps
Nausea
Nervousness
Rapid heartrate (tachycardia)
Redness around the nose
Runny nose
Seizures
Shakiness
Sleep problems (insomnia)
Thirst
Tremors
Trouble breathing
Uncontrollable shaking of a part of the body
Vomiting
Note: An overdose of Symbicort (budesonide and fomoterol) can be fatal

Tegretol (carbamazepine)

Abnormal movements
Blurred vision
Coma
Coordination problems
Difficulty breathing
Difficulty urination
Dizziness
Drowsiness
Fainting
Fast heartbeat
Feeling light-headed
Irregular or slowed breathing
Large (dilated) pupils (the dark circles in the middle of each eye)
Loss of consciousness

Muscle twitching
Nausea
Rapid or pounding heartbeat (tachycardia)
Restlessness
Seizures
Shakiness
Shaking of a part of the body that you cannot control
Shallow breathing
Shock
Slurred speech
Staggering walk
Tremors
Twitching
Unconsciousness
Unsteadiness
Unusual body movements or postures
Urinating less or not at all
Vomiting

Tenex (guanfacine)

Blurred vision
Confusion
Diarrhea
Dizziness
Drowsiness
Extreme drowsiness
Fainting
Fast, slow, or uneven heartbeats
Feeling like you might pass out
Irritability
Lack of energy
Light-headedness
Loss of appetite
Nausea

Seeing halos around lights or objects
Seizures
Severe skin rash
Slow heart rate
Sluggish feeling
Smaller (constricted) pupils (black circles in the middle of each eye)
Vomiting
Weakness

Tofranil (imipramine)

Agitation
Blue lips or fingernails
Blurred vision
Breathing slowed and labored
Coma
Confusion
Constipation
Convulsions
Enlarged pupils in the eye (pupils are the dark circles in the center of the eyes)
Delirium (decline in attention and mental process)
Dizziness
Drowziness
Dry mouth
Extreme drowsiness
Fainting
Fatigue
Feeling light-headed
Hallucinations (see or hearing things others don't)
Irregular heartbeat
Low blood pressure
Muscle spasms
Muscles becoming rigid

Muscles swelling
Restlessness
Seizures
Shock
Shortness of breath
Skin flushing
Stupor (lack of alertness)
Sweating
Uncoordinated movement
Uneven heartbeats
Urinary hesitancy (trouble releasing urine from the body)
Vomiting

An overdose of Tofranil (imipramine) can be fatal.

Toprol (metoprolol)

Abnormal heart rhythms (arrhythmia)
Bluish-colored fingernails
Confusion
Death
Decrease in breathing
Decrease in heart rate (bradycardia)
Difficulty breathing
Difficulty swallowing
Dizziness
Extremely low blood pressure
Fainting
Heart failure
Low blood sugar (hypoglycemia)
Nausea
Shortness of breath
Slow or uneven heartbeats
Swelling of hands

Swelling of the feet, ankles or lower legs
Tiredness
Vomiting
Weakness
Wheezing

Valium (diazepam)

The most obvious feature or characteristic of this overdose is falling into a deep sleep or "coma" while still being able to breathe adequately

Bluish colored lips or fingernails
Blurred vision
Breathing labored
Breathing that stops
Coma
Confusion
Depression
Dizziness
Double vision
Drowsiness
Extreme drowsiness
Excitability
Fainting
Hiccups
Limp or weak muscles
Muscle weakness
Rapid side-to-side movement of the eyes (nystagmus)
Rash
Shallow breathing
Stomach upset
Stupor (lack of alertness)
Tiredness
Tremor

Uncoordinated movements
Weakness

Valtrex (valacyclovir)

Aggressive behavior
Back pain
Confusion
Decreased urine output
Drowsiness
Hallucinations
Headache
Kidney problems or kidney failure
Loss of consciousness
Nervous system problems
Seizures
Speech problems
Tremors
Unsteady or shaky movements

Viagra (sildenafil)

Blurred vision
Chest pain
Cyanopsia (a condition which causes everything to appear
to be tinted blue)
Dizziness
Erection lasting four hours or more
Fainting
Feeling faint
Feeling light-headed
Heart attack
Irregular heartbeat
Nausea
Prolonged erection

Rapid pulse
Sensitivity to light
Severe dizziness
Sudden hearing loss
Sudden indigestion
Swelling of the ankles or legs
Vision problems
Vomiting

Vicodin (hydrocodone and acetaminophen)

As a combination product composed of acetaminophen and hydrocodone the overdose signs and symptoms of Vicodin include those attributable to each drug individual and to the combination.

Bleeding
Blue lips
Cardiac arrest (heart attack)
Cold, clammy or blue skin
Coma
Confusion
Dark urine
Death
Diarrhea
Difficulty breathing
Excessive Sleepiness
Extreme drowsiness leading to a coma
Extreme fatigue
Extreme tiredness
Fainting
Flu-like symptoms
Irritability
Liver failure
Loss of appetite

Loss of consciousness
Low blood pressure (hypotension)
Low blood sugar (hypoglycemia)
Muscle weakness
Narrowed pupils
Nausea
No breathing
Pain in the upper stomach
Pain in the upper right part of the stomach
Pinpoint pupils
Seizures
Shallow breathing
Slow heart rate (bradycardia)
Slow, shallow or stopped breathing
Stomach pain
Sweating
Unusual bleeding or bruising
Vomiting
Weakness
Weak pulse
Widened pupils
Yellowing of the skin or the whites of your eyes (jaundice)

Overdose symptoms of Vicodin include death.

Vistaril (hydroxyzine)

Blurred vision
Coma
Convulsions
Delirium
Depression
Difficulty urinating
Disorientation

Dizziness
Drowsiness
Dry mouth, nose and throat
Excitation
Extreme drowsiness
Feeling like you might pass out
Flushed skin
Hallucinations (seeing or hearing things others do not)
Low blood pressure
Nausea
Nervousness
Palpitations (sensation of an abnormality of one's heartbeat)
Rapid heart rate
Shortness of breath
Sleeping difficulties
Tremor
Uncoordinated movements
Unsteadiness
Vomiting

Vivactil (protriptyline)

An overdose of Vivactil (protriptyline) can be fatal.
Agitation
Blurred vision
Coma
Confusion
Convulsions
Dilated (widened) pupils (the dark circle in the center of each eye)
Disturbed concentration
Drowsiness
Extreme drowsiness
Fainting

Fast, irregular heartbeat
Feeling hot
Feeling cold
Fever
Hallucinations (hearing or seeing things others don't)
Hyperactive reflexes (hyperactive means highly or excessively active)
Irregular heartbeat
Loss of consciousness
Low body temperature
Muscle stiffness
Problems concentrating
Seizures
Shallow breathing
Slow breathing
Sporadic hallucinations
Stupor
Vomiting

Vyvanse (lisdexamfetamine)

Aggressiveness
Coma
Confusion
Convulsions
Cramps
Dark colored urine
Death
Depression
Diarrhea
Fainting
Fast breathing
Fast heart rate
Feeling light-headed
Feelings of panic

Fever
Flu-like symptoms
Hallucinations (seeing or hearing others do not)
High blood pressure (hypertension)
Irregular heart rhythm (arrhythmia)
Low blood pressure (hypotension)
Muscle pain
Muscle tenderness
Muscle twitches
Muscle weakness or aching
Nausea
Overactive reflexes
Panic
Rapid breathing
Restlessness
Seizures
Shakiness
Stomach cramps
Stomach pain
Tiredness
Tremors
Uncontrollable shaking of a part of the body
Uneven heartbeats
Vomiting
Weakness
Overdose symptoms of Vyvanse include death.

Wellbutrin and Wellbutrin XL (bupropion)

Blurred vision
Breathing problems
Coma
Confusion
Death

Difficulty breathing
Difficulty swallowing
Dizziness
Fainting
Fast heartbeat
Fever
Hallucinations (seeing or hearing things that others don't)
Heart attack
Irregular heart rhythms
Jitteriness
Lack of energy
Light-headedness
Loss of consciousness
Low blood pressure (hypotension)
Muscle damage
Muscle stiffness
Muscle tension
Muscle pain
Rapid heart rate (tachycardia)
Rapid or pounding heartbeat
Seizures
Shakiness
Shallow breathing
Sweating
Uneven heartbeat
Upset stomach
Weakness
Overdose symptoms of Wellbutrin and Wellbutrin XL
include death.

Xanax (alprazolam)

Appearance of being drunk
Breathing problems
Coma
Confusion
Coordination problems
Death
Difficulty breathing
Dizziness
Drowsiness
Extreme drowsiness
Fainting
Feeling light-headed
Impaired coordination
Intoxicated appearance
Loss of balance
Loss of coordination
Muscle weakness
Sleepiness
Slow heart beat
Slow reflexes
Slowed reaction time
Talking Difficulty
Walking difficulty

An overdose of Xanax can be fatal.

Zithromax (azithromycin)

Diarrhea
Loss of strength
Nausea
Stomach discomfort
Vomiting

Zocor (simvastatin)

Diarrhea
Indigestion
Nausea
Stomach distress

Zoloft (sertraline)

Agitation
Coma
Confusion
Death
Delirium
Diarrhea
Dizziness
Drowsiness
Enlarged pupils (the dark circles in the center of each eye)
Excessive tiredness
Excitement
Fainting
Hair loss
Hallucinations (seeing or hearing things that others do not)
High blood pressure (hypertension)
Hyperactivity (abnormally high level of movement)
Increased heart rate (tachycardia)
Rapid, pounding or irregular heartbeat
Seizures
Sex drive or ability changes
Shakiness
Sleeping difficulties – difficulty falling asleep or staying asleep

Slow heart rate (bradycardia)
Tremors
Unconsciousness
Uncontrollable shaking of a part of the body
Vomiting

Zyban (bupropion)

Blurred vision
Breathing problems
Coma
Confusion
Death
Difficulty breathing
Difficulty swallowing
Dizziness
Fainting
Fast heartbeat
Fever
Hallucinations (seeing or hearing things that others don't)
Heart attack
Irregular heart rhythms
Jitteriness
Lack of energy
Light-headedness
Loss of consciousness
Low blood pressure (hypotension)
Muscle damage
Muscle stiffness
Muscle tension
Muscle pain
Rapid heart rate (tachycardia)
Rapid or pounding heartbeat
Seizures
Shakiness

Shallow breathing
Sweating
Uneven heartbeat
Upset stomach
Weakness
Overdose symptoms of Zyban may include death.

Zyprexa (olanzapine)

Aggression
Agitation
Cardiac arrest
Chest pain
Coma
Convulsions
Death
Decreased breathing
Decreased consciousness
Drowsiness
Fainting
Fast heart rate (tachycardia)
High blood pressure (hypertension)
Jerky muscle movements
Loss of consciousness
Low blood pressure (hypotension)Seizures
Seizures
Slurred Speech
Sudden movements you can't control
Trouble breathing
Uncontrolled muscle movements
Vomiting

Alphabetical by Generic Name

Alprazolam (Xanax)

Appearance of being drunk
Breathing problems
Coma
Confusion
Coordination problems
Death
Difficulty breathing
Dizziness
Drowsiness
Extreme drowsiness
Fainting
Feeling light-headed
Impaired coordination
Intoxicated appearance
Loss of balance
Loss of coordination
Muscle weakness
Sleepiness
Slow heart beat
Slow reflexes
Slowed reaction time
Talking Difficulty
Walking difficulty

An overdose of Xanax can be fatal.

Amitriptyline (Elavil)

Agitation
Blurred vision
Changes in heart rhythm
Cold body temperature
Coma
Confusion
Convulsions
Drowsiness
Fainting
Feeling cold
Feeling hot
Feeling light-headed
Fever
Hallucinating (seeing things or hearing voices that do not exist)
Hypotension (very low blood pressure)
Irregular heartbeats
Muscle stiffness
Problems concentrating
Restlessness
Rigid muscles
Seizures
Sleepiness
Sweating
Uneven heartbeats
Vomiting

An overdose of Elavil can be fatal.

Amlodipine

Chest pain
Dizziness
Fainting
Feelings of a rapidly or forcefully beating heart
Light-headedness
Low blood pressure
Rapid heartbeat (tachycardia)
Severe dizziness
Warmth or tingly feeling
Weakness

Amoxicillin

Behavior changes
Black-out
Convulsions
Confusion
Diarrhea
Loss of feeling in fingers or toes
Muscle spasms
Muscle weakness
Nausea
Pain
Pain in fingers or toes
Possible kidney failure with a large overdose
Severe skin rash
Shortness of breath
Stomach cramps
Twitching
Urinating less than usual
Seizures
Vomiting

Amphetamine and Dextroamphetamine (Adderall and Adderall XR)

An overdose of (amphetamine and dextroamphetamine) Adderall can be fatal. If you think you or someone you know may have overdosed get help immediately even if you are unaware of any symptoms.

Aggressiveness / Aggressive behavior
Behavior Changes
Blurred vision
Coma
Confusion
Convulsions
Dark red or cola-colored urine
Dehydration
Delusions
Depression
Diarrhea
Dizziness
Fainting
Fast heartbeats
Feeling light-headed
Feelings of panic
Fever or flu symptoms
Hallucinations (seeing things and hearing voices that do not exist)
Heart attack
Increased blood pressure
Lower abdominal pain
Muscle weakness
Muscle Twitches
Nausea
Numbness
Numbing of fingertips
Panic

Personality changes
Rapid breathing
Restlessness
Seizures (convulsions)
Stomach pain
Stroke
Sweating
Swelling of hands, feet or ankles
Tiredness
Tremor
Trouble concentrating
Uncontrollable shaking of a part of the body
Uneven or irregular heartbeats
Unexplained muscle pain or tenderness
Upset stomach
Vomiting
Weakness

Chronic abuse can manifest itself as psychosis

Aripiprazole (Abilify)

Aggression
Agitation
Changes in heartbeat
Confusion
Coma
Difficulty breathing
Drowsiness
Fainting
Feeling light-headed
High blood pressure
Irregular heart rhythm
Lethargy (sleepy, drowsy, out of sorts, sluggish, apathetic –

it can also mean a state of unconsciousness resembling a deep sleep)
Loss of consciousness
Low Blood Potassium (your doctor can test for this)
Movements you cannot control
Nausea
Pneumonia
Seizures
Shakiness
Slowed Heart Rate
Unusual mental changes
Vomiting
Weakness
Widened Pupils (the black circles in the middle of the eyes)

Atenolol (Tenormin)

Blurred vision
Breathing problems (slow or shallow breathing)
Chest pain
Confusion
Congestive heart failure (a life-threatening condition where the heart can no longer pump enough blood to the rest of the body)
Difficulty breathing
Dizziness
Fainting
Headache
Hunger (sudden hunger)
Lack of energy
Low blood sugar
Low blood pressure
Numbness or tingling of the mouth
Pale color

Pounding in chest
Rapid heartbeat
Seizures
Severe dizziness
Severe weakness
Slow heartbeat
Sluggishness
Sweating
Tiredness (excessive)
Very slow heartbeat (unusually slow heartbeat)
Weakness
Wheezing

Atomoxetine (Strattera)

Abnormal behavior
Agitation
Blurred vision
Dilated (wide) pupils (the drak circles in the center of each eye)
Drowsiness
Dry mouth
Fast heart rate
Hallucinations (seeing or hearing things others do not)
Hyperactivity
Increase in activity or talking
Irregular heart rhythms (arrhythmias)
Sleepiness
Stomach or intestinal problems
Unusual behavior

Atorvastatin (Lipitor)

The symptoms of Lipitor overdose are not known. If you suspect you have taken more Lipitor than prescribed call poison control or your doctor right away.

Atorvastatin and Amlodipine (Caduet)

Dizziness
Fainting
Feeling light-headed
Rapid heartbeat
Redness
Severe warmth
Tingly feeling
Tingly under your skin

Azithromycin (Zithromax)

Diarrhea
Loss of strength
Nausea
Stomach discomfort
Vomiting

Bevacizumab Injection (Avastin)

Severe headache

Budesonide and Fomoterol (Symbicort)

Cardiac arrest (heart attack)
Chest pain
Convulsions
Death
Difficulty falling asleep or staying asleep
Dizziness
Dry mouth
Excessive tiredness
Fainting
Fast, pounding or irregular heartbeat
Fatigue
Headache
Heart palpitations (feeling of a rapidly or forcefully beating heart)
High blood pressure (hypertension)
High blood sugar (hyperglycemia)
Increased salivation
Low blood pressure (hypotension)
Low blood potassium (hypokalemia)
Muscle cramps
Nausea
Nervousness
Rapid heartrate (tachycardia)
Redness around the nose
Runny nose
Seizures
Shakiness
Sleep problems (insomnia)
Thirst
Tremors
Trouble breathing
Uncontrollable shaking of a part of the body
Vomiting

Note: An overdose of Symbicort (budesonide and fomoterol) can be fatal

Bupropion
(Wellbutrin, Wellbutrin XL, Zyban)

Blurred vision
Breathing problems
Coma
Confusion
Death
Difficulty breathing
Difficulty swallowing
Dizziness
Fainting
Fast heartbeat
Fever
Hallucinations (seeing or hearing things that others don't)
Heart attack
Irregular heart rhythms
Jitteriness
Lack of energy
Light-headedness
Loss of consciousness
Low blood pressure (hypotension)
Muscle damage
Muscle stiffness
Muscle tension
Muscle pain
Rapid heart rate (tachycardia)
Rapid or pounding heartbeat
Seizures
Shakiness
Shallow breathing

Sweating
Uneven heartbeat
Upset stomach
Weakness
Overdose symptoms of bupropion include death.

Buspirone (BuSpar)

Blurred vision
Dizziness
Drowsiness
Nausea
Stomach pain
Unusually small pupils
Upset stomach
Very deep sleep
Vomiting

Carbamazepine (Carbatrol, Tegretol)

Abnormal movements
Blurred vision
Difficulty urinating (urinating less or not at all)
Dizziness
Drowsiness
Fainting
Fast heartbeat
Feeling light-headed
Irregular or slowed breathing
Muscle twitching
Nausea
Rapid or pounding heartbeat
Restlessness
Shaking of a part of your body that you cannot control

Shallow breathing
Seizures
Slurred speech
Staggering walk
Tremors
Unconsciousness
Unsteadiness
Vomiting

Citlopram (Celexa)

Amnesia (memory loss)
Blue skin
Coma
Confusion
Death
Dizziness
Drowsiness
Memory loss
Muscle pain
Nausea
Rapid breathing
Rapid, irregular or pounding heartbeat
Seizures
Sweating
Tremor (Shakiness)
Trouble breathing
Uncontrollable shaking of a part of the body
Vomiting

Clomipramine (Anafranil)

Agitation
Blue discoloration of the skin
Blue lips or fingernails
Blurred vision
Cardiac arrest (heart attack)
Coma
Confusion
Congestive heart failure
Convulsions
Death
Drowsiness
Fainting
Fast or uneven heartbeat
Fever
Hallucinations
Kidney failure
Light-headedness
Loss of coordination
Low blood pressure (hypotension)
Muscle stiffness
Rapid heart rate (tachycardia)
Restlessness
Seizures
Shortness of breath
Slowed breathing
Stiff muscles
Severe Sweating
Swelling
Unusual body movements
Urination changes (urinating less or more than usual)
Vomiting
Widened pupils (the pupil is the dark circle in the center of the eye)

An overdose of Anafranil (clomipramine) can be fatal. If you think you or someone you know may have overdosed get help immediately even if you are unaware of any symptoms.

Clonazepam (Klonopin)

Alterations in mental status
Appearance of being drunk
Coma
Confusion
Difficulty breathing
Difficulty talking
Difficulty walking
Diminished reflexes
Dizziness
Drowsiness
Fainting
Muscle weakness
Slow heartbeat
Somnolence (a state of sleepiness, drowsiness)

If you suspect you suspect you have taken an overdose of this medication seek emergency medical attention right away. In some circumstances, especially when this drug is mixed with alcohol or other sedating drugs, overdose can lead to the person being unable to breathe and dying.

Klonopin can be habit-forming and can lose its effectiveness as you build a tolerance to it. This can lead to unintentional overdose.

Clonidine (Catapres)

Anxiety
Blurred vision
Buzzing in your ears
Chest pain
Cold feeling
Cold, pale skin
Coma
Confusion
Decreased reflexes
Difficulty breathing
Drowsiness
Fainting
Feeling light-headed
High blood pressure
High blood pressure followed by low blood pressure
Irritability
Low blood pressure
Low body temperature
Seizures
Severe headache
Shallow or slow breathing
Shivering
Shortness of breath
Slow heart rate
Slurred speech
Smaller pupils - also called Pinpoint pupils (black circles in
the middle of your eyes)
Tiredness
Weakness

Clopidogrel (Plavix)

Blood in your stools
Blood in your vomit
Difficulty breathing
Exhaustion
Shortness of breath
Unusual bruising or bleeding
Vomiting

Clozapine (Clozaril)

If overdose is suspected if even the symptoms are not on this list call 911 and get to an emergency room immediately.

Change in heartbeat
Coma
Delerium
Difficult or slow breathing
Dizziness
Drowsines
Excessive salivation
Fainting
Fast or irregular heartbeat
Loss of consciousness
Seizures
Slow breathing
Severe or persistent dizziness
Severe or persistent drowsiness

Desipramine (Norpramin)

An overdose of desipramine (Norpramin) can be fatal.

Agitation
Blurred vision
Change in heart rhythm
Coma
Confusion
Convulsions
Death
Dilated (wide open) pupils (the dark circle in the middle of each eye)
Disturbed concentration
Drowsiness
Extremely low blood pressure
Feeling cold
Feeling hot
Hallucinations (seeing or hearing things that do not exist)
High fever
Irregular heart rate
Low body temperature (hypothermia)
Muscle stiffness
Muscle tension
Overactive reflexes
Rigid muscles
Seizures
Stupor
Trouble concentrating
Uneven heartbeats
Very low blood pressure
Vomiting

Desvenlafaxine (Pristiq)

Abdominal pain
Agitation
Constipation
Diarrhea
Dizziness
Drowsiness
Dry Mouth
Fast heartbeat (tachycardia)
Headache
Nausea
Numbness
Pain, burning, numbness or tingling in any part of the body
Seizures
Slow heart rate
Tingly Feeling
Tremor
Unusual sensations, such as burning or tingling
Vomiting

Dextroamphetamine (Dexedrine)

Abdominal cramps
Aggressive behavior
Blurred Vision
Coma
Confusion
Convulsions
Depression
Diarrhea
Dizziness
Fainting
Fast breathing
Fatigue

Feeling light-headed
Fever
Flu symptoms
Hallucinations (seeing things or hearing voices that do not exist)
Heart rhythm abnormalities
Hyperactivity
Increased reflexes
Irregular heartbeat
Muscle pain
Muscle twitches
Muscle weakness or aching
Nausea
Panic
Rapid breathing
Restlessness
Seizures
Stomach cramps
Tiredness
Tremor
Uncontrollable shaking of a part of your body
Uneven heartbeats
Upset stomach
Urine changes (dark red or cola colored urine)
Vomiting
Weakness

An overdose of dextroamphetamine can be fatal.

Diazepam (Valium)

The most obvious feature or characteristic of this overdose is falling into a deep sleep or "coma" while still being able to breathe adequately.

Bluish colored lips or fingernails
Blurred vision
Breathing labored
Breathing that stops
Coma
Confusion
Depression
Dizziness
Double vision
Drowsiness
Extreme drowsiness
Excitability
Fainting
Hiccups
Limp or weak muscles
Muscle weakness
Rapid side-to-side movement of the eyes (nystagmus)
Rash
Shallow breathing
Stomach upset
Stupor (lack of alertness)
Tiredness
Tremor
Uncoordinated movements
Weakness

Duloxetine (Cymbalta)

Agitation
Coma
Confusion
Diarrhea
Dizziness
Drowsiness
Fainting
Fast heartbeat
Fever
Hallucinating (seeing things or hearing voices that do not exist)
Hypertension abnormally high blood pressure)
Hypotension (abnormally low blood pressure)
Light-headedness
Loss of coordination
Nausea
Seizures
Somnolence
Unresponsiveness
Vomiting

Dutasteride (Avodart)

An overdose of Avodart (dutasteride) is not expected to produce life-threatening symptoms.

Epoetin alfa injection (Epogen)

Blood clot in hemodialysis port (Hemodialysis is the removal of toxins or waste from the kidneys. Medically, a port is a small device used to put something into the body placed below the skin or in a vein)

Blue-grey color or darkening around mouth or nails
Chest pain (squeezing pressure or tightness)
Cough that won't go away
Coughing up blood
Discomfort or pain in the arms, shoulder, neck, jaw and back
Dizziness
Excessive sweating
Extreme tiredness
Extreme weakness
Fainting or loss of consciousness
Fullness in your upper stomach
Fast or irregular heartbeat
Headache (sudden and severe)
Increased blood pressure
Itching (especially after bathing)
Leg pain, tenderness, redness, warmth and / or swelling
Light-headedness
Loss of balance or coordination
Redness of the face
Seizure
Shortness of breath
Sudden confusion
Sudden trouble seeing in one or both eyes
Sudden trouble speaking or understanding speech
Sudden weakness or numbness of an arm or a leg (especially on one side of the body)

Sudden weakness or numbness of the face (especially one side)
Swelling of hands, feet, or ankles
Trouble walking (sudden)
Vision problems

Escitalopram (Lexapro)

Coma
Confusion
Convulsions
Dizziness
Drowsiness
Fast breathing
Fast pounding heartbeat
Forgetfulness
Increased heart rate (tachycardia)
Insomnia
Irregular heart rhythm (arrhythmia)
Low blood pressure (hypotension)
Nausea
Rapid heartbeat (tachycardia)
Seizures
Sweating
Tremor

Esomeprazole (Nexium)

Blurred vision
Confusion
Drowsiness
Dry mouth
Fast heartbeat
Flushing

Headache
Increased heart rate (tachycardia)
Loss of coordination
Nausea
Seizures
Shortness of breath
Sweating
Tremor

Eszopiclone (Lunesta)

A Lunesta (eszopiclone) overdose can be fatal.

Exceeding the prescribed dosage of Lunesta increases the risk of experiencing abnormal thoughts and engaging in reckless behavior. Examples include aggressive behaviors, confusion, increase in outgoingness, and suicidal ideation. In severe cases, coma and death may result. (From: http://www.ehow.com/facts_5499431_lunesta-overdose-symptoms.html)

Aggressive behaviors
Coma
Confusion
Death
Drowsiness
Increase in outgoingness
Reckless behavior
Suicidal ideation (thoughts of killing yourself)

Etanercept injection (Enbrel)

No harmful effects due to large doses of etanercept (Enbrel) have been reported. However if you suspect you have been given too much of this drug notify your doctor right away.

Fluoxetine (Prozac, Sarafem)

Agitation
Coma
Confusion
Death
Drowsiness
Enlarged pupils
Fainting
Fast heart rate (tachycardia)
Fever
Hallucinating (seeing things or hearing voices other people don't)
High blood pressure (hypertension)
Hyperactivity
Irregular heart rhythm (arrhythmia)
Low blood pressure (hypotension)
Nausea
Nervousness
Pounding heart beat
Seizures
Sleepiness
Tremor
Uncontrollable shaking of part of the body
Uneven heartbeat
Unresponsiveness
Unsteadiness
Vomiting

Fluticasone and Salmeterol (Advair Diskus)

Blurred vision
Chest pain
Difficulty falling or staying asleep
Dizziness
Dry mouth
Excessive tiredness
Fainting
Fast, pounding or irregular heartbeat
Headaches
Lack of energy
Muscle cramps or weakness
Nausea
Nervousness
Seizures
Shaking of a part of your body that you cannot control

Fluvoxamine (Luvox)

Agitation
Blurred vision
Breathing problems
Cardiac problems (heart problems)
Coma
Convulsions
Death
Diarrhea
Dizziness
Drowsiness
Enlarged pupils
Extreme drowsiness
Fainting
Fast hear rate
Hyperactivity

Irregular heart rhythms (arrhythmias)
Lack of coordination
Liver function problems
Low blood pressure (hypotension)
Low blood potassium levels (hypokalemia)
Nausea
Rapid heart rate (tachycardia)
Seizures
Shakiness
Slowed heart rate (bradycardia)
Somnolence (drowsiness, sleepiness)
Tremors
Trouble breathing
Vomiting

Furosemide (Lasix)

Confusion
Dizziness
Fainting
Fatigue
Feeling light-headed
Irregular pulse
Loss of appetite
Muscle cramps
Nausea
Ringing in your ears
Vomiting
Weakness

Guanfacine (Intuniv, Tenex)

Accidental overdose of Guanfacine (Intuniv, Tenex) is an increasing cause of poisoning in children 3 years of age and younger. (From Drugs.com)

Blurred vision
Difficult breathing
Dizziness
Drowsiness
Drowsiness leading to unresponsiveness or coma
Fainting
Feeling like you might pass out
Irritability
Lack of energy
Lightheadedness
Nausea
Seizures (possibly)
Slowed breathing
Slowed heart rate
Sluggish feeling
Smaller pupils (black circles in the middle of the eyes)
Vomiting
Weakness

Haloperidol (Haldol)

An overdose of haloperidol can be fatal.

Arrhythmia (an irregular heart rhythm)
Coma
Difficulty breathing
Drowsiness
Extreme drowsiness
Feeling like you might pass out

Loss of consciousness
Low blood pressure (hypotension)
Muscle weakness
Rigid muscles
Shakiness
Sleepiness
Slowed breathing
Stiff or weak muscles
Tremors
Uncontrolled muscle movements in your eyes
Uncontrolled muscle movements in your tongue, jaw or neck
Unusual, slowed or uncontrollable movements of any part of the body

Hydrochlorothiazide

Back pain
Confusion
Decreased urine output
Dehydration
Diarrhea
Dizziness
Drowsiness
Dry mouth
Extremely low blood pressure
Fainting
Fatigue
Headache
Increased thirst
Increased urination
Kidney Failure
Lethargy
Lightheadedness
Loss of Consciousness

Muscle pain or cramps
Muscle weakness
Nausea
Restlessness
Seizures
Slow or irregular heartbeat
Tiredness
Thirst
Weakness
Unconsciousness
Vomiting

Hydrocodone and acetaminophen (Vicodin)

As a combination product composed of acetaminophen and hydrocodone the overdose signs and symptoms of Vicodin include those attributable to each drug individual and to the combination.

Bleeding
Blue lips
Cardiac arrest (heart attack)
Cold, clammy or blue skin
Coma
Confusion
Dark urine
Death
Diarrhea
Difficulty breathing
Excessive Sleepiness
Extreme drowsiness leading to a coma
Extreme fatigue
Extreme tiredness
Fainting
Flu-like symptoms

Irritability
Liver failure
Loss of appetite
Loss of consciousness
Low blood pressure (hypotension)
Low blood sugar (hypoglycemia)
Muscle weakness
Narrowed pupils
Nausea
No breathing
Pain in the upper stomach
Pain in the upper right part of the stomach
Pinpoint pupils
Seizures
Shallow breathing
Slow heart rate (bradycardia)
Slow, shallow or stopped breathing

Hydroxyzine (Vistaril)

Blurred vision
Coma
Convulsions
Delirium
Depression
Difficulty urinating
Disorientation
Dizziness
Drowsiness
Dry mouth, nose and throat
Excitation
Extreme drowsiness
Feeling like you might pass out
Flushed skin
Hallucinations (seeing or hearing things others do not)

Low blood pressure
Nausea
Nervousness
Palpitations (sensation of an abnormality of one's heartbeat)
Rapid heart rate
Shortness of breath
Sleeping difficulties
Tremor
Uncoordinated movements
Unsteadiness
Vomiting

Ibandronate (Boniva)

Convulsions
Diarrhea
Heartburn
Indigestion
Irritability
Muscle cramps
Nausea
Numbness
Seizure
Stomach pain
Tight muscles in your face
Tingling
Ulcers
Unusual thoughts or behavior

Imipramine
(Tofranil)

Agitation
Blue lips or fingernails
Blurred vision
Breathing slowed and labored
Coma
Confusion
Constipation
Convulsions
Enlarged pupils in the eye (pupils are the dark circles in the center of the eyes)
Delirium (decline in attention and mental process)
Dizziness
Drowziness
Dry mouth
Extreme drowsiness
Fainting
Fatigue
Feeling light-headed
Hallucinations (see or hearing things others don't)
Irregular heartbeat
Low blood pressure
Muscle spasms
Muscles becoming rigid
Muscles swelling
Restlessness
Seizures
Shock
Shortness of breath
Skin flushing
Stupor (lack of alertness)
Sweating
Uncoordinated movement
Uneven heartbeats

Urinary hesitancy (trouble releasing urine from the body)
Vomiting

An overdose of Tofranil (imipramine) can be fatal.

Infliximab Injection   (Remicade)

An overdose of Remicade is not expected to produce life-threatening symptoms.

Lamatrogine (Lamictal)

Arrhythmia (irregular heartbeat)
Blurred vision
Coma
Coordination problems
Crossed eyes
Death
Fainting
Feeling light-headed
Headache
Increased seizures
Involuntary eye movements
Loss of balance or coordination
Loss of consciousness
Seizures
Unconsciousness

Lisdexamfetamine (Vyvanse)

Aggressiveness
Coma
Confusion
Convulsions
Cramps
Dark colored urine
Death
Depression
Diarrhea
Fainting
Fast breathing
Fast heart rate
Feeling light-headed
Feelings of panic
Fever
Flu-like symptoms
Hallucinations (seeing or hearing others do not)
High blood pressure (hypertension)
Irregular heart rhythm (arrhythmia)
Low blood pressure (hypotension)
Muscle pain
Muscle tenderness
Muscle twitches
Muscle weakness or aching
Nausea
Overactive reflexes
Panic
Rapid breathing
Restlessness
Seizures
Shakiness
Stomach cramps
Stomach pain
Tiredness

Tremors
Uncontrollable shaking of a part of the body
Uneven heartbeats
Vomiting
Weakness
Overdose symptoms of Vyvanse (lisdexamfetamine) include death.

Lisinopril (Prinvil, Zestril)

Dizziness
Extreme dizziness
Fainting
Fatigue
Light-headedness
Weakness

Lithium Carbonate (Eskalith, Lithium, Lithobid)

Blurred vision
Confusion
Convulsions
Diarrhea
Drowsiness
Increased thirst
Increased urine output
Loss of appetite
Loss of coordination
Low blood pressure
Muscle twitching
Muscle weakness
Nausea
Rash
Ringing in your ears

Seizures
Sluggishness
Tremor
Vomiting

Lorazepam (Ativan)

Appearance of being drunk
Breathing difficulty
Coma
Confusion
Difficulty talking
Drowsiness
Extreme drowsiness
Fainting
Hypnotic state
Low blood pressure
Mental confusion
Muscle weakness
Reduced muscle tone
Shallow breathing
Sleepiness
Slow heart beat
Stupor
Tiredness
Unsteady walk
Weakness

Maprotiline (Ludiomil)

Agitation
Blue fingernails
Blue lips
Confusion
Convulsions
Dizziness
Drowsiness (extreme)
Extreme drowsiness
Fast heart rate
Fever
Irregular heartbeat
Large pupils
Muscle weakness
Muscle stiffness
Poor memory
Restlessness
Seizures
Trouble breathing
Vomiting

Metformin (Glucophage)

An overdose of metformin (Glucophage) can be life-threatening. If you suspect an overdose has occurred get emergency help immediately.

An overdose of metformin may cause a life-threatening condition called lactic acidosis.

Get emergency medical help if you have any of these symptoms of lactic acidosis: weakness, increasing sleepiness, slow heart rate, cold feeling, muscle pain, shortness of breath, stomach pain, feeling light-headed, and fainting.

Other overdose signs and symptoms include:

Abnormally fast or slow heartbeat
Blurry vision
Cold sweats
Coma
Confusion
Convulsions
Death
Decreased appetite
Deep, rapid breathing
Difficulty speaking
Discomfort
Dizziness
Drowsiness
Extreme tiredness
Fainting
Feeling cold
Flushing of the skin
Headache
Hunger
Irritability
Light-headedness
Loss of consciousness
Loss of coordination
Muscle pain
Nausea
Shakiness
Shortness of breath
Seizures

Stomach pain
Sweating
Tremors
Vomiting
Weakness

Methylphenidate (Concerta, Ritalin, Metadate, Methylin)

Aggressiveness
Agitation
Blurred vision
Confusion
Dry mouth and nose
Fainting
Fast breathing
Fast heartbeat
Fast, pounding or irregular heartbeat
Fever
Flushing
Hallucinations (seeing or hearing things that are not really there)
Headache
Hyperactivity (trouble sitting still)
Inappropriate happiness
Large pupils
Loss of consciousness
Muscle pains
Muscle twitches
Seizures (convulsions)
Shakiness
Sweating
Tremors
Uncontrollable shaking of a body part

Widening of pupils (the black circles in the middle of your eyes)
Vomiting

Metoprolol (Toprol)

Abnormal heart rhythms (arrhythmia)
Bluish-colored fingernails
Confusion
Death
Decrease in breathing
Decrease in heart rate (bradycardia)
Difficulty breathing
Difficulty swallowing
Dizziness
Extremely low blood pressure
Fainting
Heart failure
Low blood sugar (hypoglycemia)
Nausea
Shortness of breath
Slow or uneven heartbeats
Swelling of hands
Swelling of the feet, ankles or lower legs
Tiredness
Vomiting
Weakness
Wheezing

Mirtapazine (Remeron)

Confusion
Death
Disorientation
Drowsiness
Memory problems
Poor memory
Rapid heart rate (tachycardia)
Note: Possible overdose symptoms of Remeron
(Mirtapazine) include death.

Molindone (Moban)

Seek emergency medical attention immediately if you think
you have used too much of this drug.

Agitation
Coma
Convulsions
Death
Difficulty breathing
Dizziness
Drowziness
Fainting
Fever
Increased salivation
Irregular heart rhythm (arrhythmia)
Loss on consciousness
Low blood pressure (hypotension)
Muscle stiffness
Muscle twitching
Restlessness
Seizures

Slurred speech
Trouble swallowing
Unconsciousness
Unusual body or facial movements
Unusual, slowed or uncontrollable movements of any part
of the body

Memetasone nasal inhalation (Nasonex)

An overdose of this medication is not likely to occur. If you
do suspect an overdose contact poison control.

Nasonex is a topical steroid and long-term use of high
steroid doses can lead to symptoms such as thinning skin,
easy bruising, changes in the shape or location of body fat
(especially in your face, neck, back, and waist), increased
acne or facial hair, menstrual problems, impotence, or loss
of interest in sex.

Montelukast (Singulair)

Agitation
Dizziness
Headache
restlessness
Sleepiness
Stomach pain
Thirst
Vomiting

Nortriptyline (Pamelor)

Agitation
Blurred vision
Confusion
Coma
Convulsions
Dilated pupils (the pupils are the dark circles in the middle of the eyes)
Disturbed concentration
Dizziness
Drowsiness
Excessive reflexes
Extreme drowsiness
Extremely high fever
Fainting
Fatigue
Feeling hot
Feeling cold
Fever
Fluid in the lungs
Hallucinations (seeing or hearing things that do not exist)
Heart failure
Irregular heartbeat
Low blood pressure
Low body temperature
Restlessness
Rigid muscles
Seizures
Shock
Stiff muscles
Stupor
Vomiting
Widened pupils (the pupils are the dark circles in the middle of the eyes)

An overdose of nortriptyline (Pamelor) can be fatal.

Olanzapine (Zyprexa)

Aggression
Agitation
Cardiac arrest
Chest pain
Coma
Convulsions
Death
Decreased breathing
Decreased consciousness
Drowsiness
Fainting
Fast heart rate (tachycardia)
High blood pressure (hypertension)
Jerky muscle movements
Loss of consciousness
Low blood pressure (hypotension)Seizures
Seizures
Slurred Speech
Sudden movements you can't control
Trouble breathing
Uncontrolled muscle movements
Vomiting

Omeprazole

Blurred vision
Confusion
Decreased body temperature
Drowsiness
Dry mouth
Fast or pounding heartbeat)
Flushing (sudden reddening and feeling of warmth)
Headaches
Nausea
Rapid heart rate (tachycardia)
Seizures
Shortness of breath
Sweating
Vomiting

Oxycodone (Oxycontin)

Blue color of skin, fingernals, lips, area around the mouth
Cardiac arrest (heart attack)
Cold, clammy skin
Coma
Confusion
Death
Difficulty breathing
Dizziness
Excessive sleepiness
Extreme drowsiness, leading to coma
Fainting
Increase in size (dilated) of pupils (the black circles in the middle of the eye)
Loss of consciousness
Low blood pressure (hypotension)

Seizures
Shallow breathing
Slow breathing
Slowed or stopped breathing
Slow heart rate (bradycardia)
Small pupils (the black circles in the middle of the eye)
Tiredness
Weak, limp muscles
Weakness

An overdose of Oxycontin (oxycodone) can be fatal.

Paroxetine (Paxil)

Aggressive behavior
Agitation
Blurred vision
Coma
Confusion
Dark red or brown urine
Death
Decreased urination
Diarrhea
Difficulty urinating
Difficulty walking
Dizziness
Drowsiness
Enlarged pupils
Extreme tiredness
Fainting
Fast, pounding, irregular, or slow heartbeat
Fever
Flu-like symptoms
Frenzied, abnormally excited mood

High blood pressure (hypertension)
Hyperactivity
Irregular heart rhythm (arrhythmia)
Kidney failure
Lack of energy
Liver problems, including hepatitis
Loss of appetite
Low blood pressure (hypotension)
Muscle pain, stiffness, or weakness
Nausea
Pain in the upper right part of the stomach
Rapid heartbeat (tachycardia)
Seizures
Shakiness
Slow heart rate (bradycardia)
Sudden muscle twitching or jerking that you cannot control
Sweating
Tremor
Uncontrollable shaking of a part of the body
Unusual bruising or bleeding
Vomiting
Yellowing of the skin and eyes

Pegfilgrastim (Neulasta)

Overdose symptoms for this drug are not known.

Pimozide (Orap)

Blank facial expression
Coma
Death
Difficulty breathing
Dizziness
Drowsiness
Fast heartbeat
Restlessness
Shuffling walk
Uncontrollable movements
Unusual, slowed or uncontrollable movement of any part of the body

An overdose of Orap (pimozide) can be fatal.

Pioglitazone (Actos)

Since there have been very few reported cases of people who have overdosed on Actos (Pioglitazone), the full effects of an Actos overdose are not known. But any medication taking in excess can cause serious problems. If you suspect you have taken too much Actos do not wait for symptoms but call poison control and 911 right away.

Pregabalin (Lyrica)

It is unknown exactly what to expect from a Lyrica overdose, but patients who are suspected of overdosing should seek emergency medical attention or contact the local Poison Control Center by calling 1-800-222-1222 or call local emergency services at 911.

Protriptyline (Vivactil)

An overdose of Vivactil (protriptyline) can be fatal.
Agitation
Blurred vision
Coma
Confusion
Convulsions
Dilated (widened) pupils (the dark circle in the center of each eye)
Disturbed concentration
Drowsiness
Extreme drowsiness
Fainting
Fast, irregular heartbeat
Feeling hot
Feeling cold
Fever
Hallucinations (hearing or seeing things others don't)
Hyperactive reflexes (hyperactive means highly or excessively active)
Irregular heartbeat
Loss of consciousness
Low body temperature
Muscle stiffness
Problems concentrating
Seizures

Shallow breathing
Slow breathing
Sporadic hallucinations
Stupor
Vomiting

Quetiapine (Seroquel)

Coma
Death
Dizziness
Drowsiness
Extreme Drowsiness
Fainting
Fast heartbeat (tachycardia)
Feeling light-headed
Irregular heart rhythm (arrhythmia)
Low blood potassium (hypokalemia)
Low blood pressure (hypotension)
Note: Possible overdose symptoms of Seroquel include death.

Raloxifene (Evista)

Coordination problems
Diarrhea
Dizziness
Flushing
Leg cramps
Loss of coordination
Rash
Shakiness
Tremor
Vomiting

Risperidone (Risperdal)

Blurred vision
Death
Dizziness
Drowsiness
Fainting
Fast, pounding or irregular heartbeat
Feeling light-headed
Fever
Irregular heart rhythm
Muscle spasms
Restless muscle movements in your eyes, tongue, jaw or neck
Seizures
Shakiness
Sweating
Uncontrollable movements of the arms, hands eyes, tongue, jaw or neck
Uncontrollable muscle contractions or other unusual body movements
Upset stomach
Note: Possible overdose symptoms of Risperdal (Risperidone) include death.

Rosaglitizone (Avandia)

Signs of low blood sugar including:
Hunger
Confusion
Irritability

Drowsiness
Weakness
Dizziness
Tremors
Sweating
Rapid heartbeat
Seizure
Convulsions
Fainting
Coma

Rosuvastatin (Crestor)

No specific information is available regarding overdose symptoms connected with taking Crestor (Rosuvastatin). As with any other medication if you suspect you have taken an overdose of Crestor (Rosuvastatin) seek medical attention immediately.

Sertraline (Zoloft)

Agitation
Coma
Confusion
Death
Delirium
Diarrhea
Dizziness
Drowsiness
Enlarged pupils (the dark circles in the center of each eye)
Excessive tiredness
Excitement
Fainting

Hair loss
Hallucinations (seeing or hearing things that others do not)
High blood pressure (hypertension)
Hyperactivity (abnormally high level of movement)
Increased heart rate (tachycardia)
Rapid, pounding or irregular heartbeat
Seizures
Sex drive or ability changes
Shakiness
Sleeping difficulties – difficulty falling asleep or staying asleep
Slow heart rate (bradycardia)
Tremors
Unconsciousness
Uncontrollable shaking of a part of the body
Vomiting

Sildenafil (Viagra)

Blurred vision
Chest pain
Cyanopsia (a condition which causes everything to appear to be tinted blue)
Dizziness
Erection lasting four hours or more
Fainting
Feeling faint
Feeling light-headed
Heart attack
Irregular heartbeat
Nausea
Prolonged erection
Rapid pulse
Sensitivity to light
Severe dizziness

Sudden hearing loss
Sudden indigestion
Swelling of the ankles or legs
Vision problems
Vomiting

Simvastatin (Zocor)

Diarrhea
Indigestion
Nausea
Stomach distress

Sitagliptin (Januvia)

Agitation
Coma
Confusion
Convulsions
Dizziness
Drowsiness
Fainting
Fast heartbeat
Headache
Hunger (as a sign of low blood sugar)
Irritability
Seizures
Sweating
Tremors
Vision changes
Weakness

If you think you may have taken more than the prescribed amount of Januvia seek emergency medical attention right away.

Tadalafil (Cialis)

Chest Pain
Erection that lasts longer than 4 hours
Fainting
Feeling light-headed
Flushing
Headache
Heartburn
Indigestion
Irregular heartbeat
Nausea
Pain in the back
Pain in the muscles or any limb
Stuffy or runny nose

Tamsulosin (Flomax)

Blurred vision
Cold and clammy skin
Coma
Dizziness
Extreme dizziness
Fainting
Headache
Light-headedness
Loss of consciousness
Upset stomach

Weak, fast pulse
Weakness

Thioridazine (Mellaril)

An overdose of Mellaril (methylphenidate) can be fatal. If you suspect an overdose, seek medical help immediately.

Agitation
Blurred vision
Coma
Confusion
Constipation
Convulsions
Decreased urination
Difficulty breathing
Difficulty urinating
Difficulty walking
Drooling
Drowsiness
Dry mouth
Dry skin
Extreme dizziness
Fainting
Fast heartbeat
Feeling hot or feeling cold
Fever
High body temperature
Intestinal obstruction
Irregular heartbeat (arrhythmias)
Loss of appetite
Loss of coordination
Low blood pressure (hypotension)
Low body temperature
Menstrual changes

Muscle spasms
Muscle stiffness
Narrowed pupil (black circle in the middle of each eye)
Nasal congestion
Pounding heartbeat
Rapid heart rate (tachycardia)
Restlessness
Seizures
Shallow breathing
Skin discoloration (blue to purple)
Slowed breathing
Slow heartbeat (bradycardia)
Slowed or unusual movements
Stiff neck or face
Stomach bloating
Stomach cramps
Stuffed nose
Swallowing difficulties
Ulcers in mouth, tongue or throat
Uncontrollable muscle movements
Vision color changes (things getting a brown tinge)
Weak breathing
Widened pupils (black circle in the middle of each eye)
Yellow eyes

Tranylcypromine (Parnate)

Agitation
Anxiety
Anxiousness

Chest pain
Cold sweats
Coma
Confusion
Dizziness
Drowsiness
Excitement
Fainting
Fast or pounding heart beat
Fatigue
Feeling light-headed
Fever
Flushing
Hallucinations (seeing or hearing things that do not exist)
Headache
High blood pressure (hypertension)
High fever
Hyperactivity
Insomnia (difficulty falling or staying asleep)
Irritability
Muscle twitching
Neck pain or stiffness
Restlessness
Sweating
Steffness
Twitching
Unclear speech
Very low blood pressure (hypotension)
Weakness

**Trazodone
(Desyrel)**

Breathing problems (breathing that slows or stops)
Changes in heartbeat

Death
Difficulty breathing
Drowsiness
Fast or pounding heartbeat
Irregular heart rhythm
Nausea
Priapism (a painful erection of the penis that does not go away)
Seizures
Vomiting

An overdose of trazodone can be fatal when it is taken with alcohol, barbiturates such as phenobarbital, or sedatives such as diazepam (Valium).

Trifluoperazine (Stelazine)

Agitation
Bloating (of stomach)
Changes in heart rate
Coma
Constipation
Convulsions
Dizziness
Drowsiness
Dry mouth
Extreme drowsiness
Fainting
Fever
High body temperature
Intestinal blockage
Irregular heartbeat (arrhythmia)
Loss of consciousness
Low blood pressure (hypotension)

Low body temperature
Restlessness
Seizures
Severe Dizziness
Sleepiness
Stomach cramps
Uncontrollable movements
Unusual body movements
Slowed or uncontrollable movements of any part of the
body
Very deep sleep

Trimipramine (Surmontil)

Abnormal dilation of the pupil (dark circle in the center of
each eye)
Agitation
Blurred vision
Changes in heart rhythm (arrhythmia)
Coma
Confusion
Convulsions
Death
Difficulty talking or articulating words
Dizziness
Drowsiness
Excitement
Extreme drowsiness
Fainting
Fatigue
Feeling light-headed
Hallucinations (seeing or hearing things that so not exist)
High fever
Low blood pressure (hypotension)
Low body temperature (hypothermia)

Muscle spasms
Muscle stiffness or tension
Seizures
Trouble breathing
Trouble concentrating
Uneven heartbeats
Vomiting

Note: An overdose of Surmontil (trimipramine) can be fatal

Valacyclovir (Valtrex)

Aggressive behavior
Back pain
Confusion
Decreased urine output
Drowsiness
Hallucinations
Headache
Kidney problems or kidney failure
Loss of consciousness
Nervous system problems
Seizures
Speech problems
Tremors
Unsteady or shaky movements

Valproic Acid (Depakote)

Coma
Confusion
Death

Decreased breathing
Deep Sleep
Drowsiness
Faint or no heartbeat
Heart block (a problem with the electrical system of the heart)
Irregular heartbeat
Loss of consciousness
Seizures
Shallow breathing
Sleepiness
Stopped breathing
Unconsciousness
Weak pulse

Valproic Acid (Depakene)

Coma
Confusion
Death
Decreased breathing
Deep Sleep
Drowsiness
Faint or no heartbeat
Heart block (a problem with the electrical system of the heart)
Irregular heartbeat
Loss of consciousness
Seizures
Shallow breathing
Sleepiness
Stopped breathing
Unconsciousness
Weak pulse

Varenicline (Chantix)

Very little information is available about overdose symptoms related to Chantix, probably because it is relatively new on the market. Since it is reasonable to expect that some overdose symptoms could be related to the usual side effects connected to this drug I will list the side effects here.

Agitation
Appetite changes (increased or decreased appetite)
Bad taste in mouth
Behavior changes
Blistering of any kind of skin rash (Report to doctor immediately – no matter how mild)
Constipation
Depression
Difficulty breathing
Drowsiness
Fever
Gas
Headache
Heartburn
Hives
Hostility
Increased appetite
Indigestion
Mood changes
Nausea
Rash
Red skin
Skin rash
Sore throat

Stomach pain
Swelling of your face, lips, tongue or throat
Thoughts of suicide
Thoughts of hurting yourself
Tired feeling
Trouble falling asleep
Trouble staying asleep
Unpleasant taste in your mouth
Unusual dream or nightmares
Weakness
Vomiting

This is not a complete list of side effects, others may occur.

Venlafaxine (Effexor and Effexor XR)

Blurred vision
Burning of hands and feet
Cold spells
Coma
Convulsions
Death
Decreased blood pressure
Dizziness
Drowsiness
Excessive tiredness (somnolence)
Hot spells
Increased heart rate
Increased size of pupil (black center of the eye)
Irregular heartbeats
Liver damage
Muscle Pain
Nausea
Numbness

Numbness of hands and feet
Seizures
Sleepiness
Slowed heart rate
Spinning sensation (vertigo)
Tingling of hands and feet
Unconsciousness
Vomiting

Ziprasidone (Geodon)

Anxiety
Dizziness
Drowsiness
Fainting
Fast or pounding heartbeat
Feeling light-headed
Fever
High blood pressure (hypertension)
Increased heart rate
Irregular heart rhythms
Muscle spasms
Problems with speech
Restless muscle movements in your eyes
Restless muscle movements in your tongue jaw or neck
Shakiness
Slurred speech
Sudden movements that you cannot control
Sweating
Twitching
Uncontrollable movements of the arms, hands or tongue
Uncontrollable shaking of a part of the body
Unusual body movements

Zoledronic Acid (Reclast)

Confusion
Depression
Difficulty breathing
Difficulty speaking
Difficulty walking
Dizziness
Double vision
Fast, pounding or irregular heartbeat
Fever
Muscle stiffness
Muscle weakness
Numbness, burning or tingling in fingers or toes
Seizures
Shortness of breath
Spasms in the muscles of your face or other areas
Sudden tightening of muscles
Trouble breathing
Uneven heartbeats
Weakness
Wheezing

Zolpidem (Ambien and Ambien CR)

Coma
Confusion
Drowsiness

Fainting
Lightheadedness
Shallow breathing
Sleepiness
Slowed breathing
Slowed heartbeat

An overdose of Ambien can be fatal when it is taken together with other medications that can cause drowsiness.

References and Sources

http://www.nlm.nih.gov/medlineplus/druginfo/meds/
http://www.ehow.com/
http://drugs.com
http://www.adderall.net/
health.yahoo.com/drug/d00168a1#d00168a1-overdose
http:// emedtv.com/
http://www.wrongdiagnosis.com/
http://www.amoxicillin.com/amoxicillin_emergency.html
http://www.medicinenet.com
health.yahoo.com/drug/d04121a1#d04121a1-overdose
www.life-extension-drugs.com/aricept.html
http://health.allrefer.com/health/thioridazine-
overdose.html
http://www.depressionforums.org/articles/778/1/Pamelor
-Nortriptyline-hydrochloride/Page1.html
http://www.nlm.nih.gov/medlineplus/ (search any drug
for overdose)

Final Notes:

Once the emergency has been taken care of you should report side effects and adverse reactions to FDA at 1-800-FDA-1088 or online at:

https://www.accessdata.fda.gov/scripts/medwatch/medwatch-online.htm

Drug brand names are registered trademarks owned by the drug's manufacturer.

Every effort has been made to ensure that the information provided is accurate, up-to-date, and complete, but no guarantee is made to that effect. This booklet is not a substitute for medical advice or reading drug labeling.

If you suspect you have taken too much of any drug call poison control immediately even if you are symptom-free.

This booklet does not include side effects and other warnings. These can be found on the labeling that came with the drug or on the FDA Medline Plus web site located here:

http://www.nlm.nih.gov/medlineplus/druginformation.html

https://www.nlm.nih.gov/medlineplus/druginfo/drug_Aa.html

http://www.nlm.nih.gov/medlineplus/druginformation.html

http://www.nlm.nih.gov/medlineplus/ (search any drug for overdose)

Other Books by Meridith

Eat, Drink, and Be Rested - The Secret Power of Food and Natural Remedied to Help You Sleep

Addictive Prescription Drugs - Find Out What's Hiding in the Fine Print

Insomnia Drugs - Side Effects and Warnings

Antidepressants - What Every Patient Needs to Know

**If you liked this book,
please leave a favorable review.**

Every Review Helps